Death in the Clinic

Practicing Bioethics

General Editor: Mark G. Kuczewski, Ph.D.
Neiswanger Institute for Bioethics and Health Policy
Loyola University Chicago

The Practicing Bioethics series provides readers with insight into the professional practices by which bioethicists, physicians, nurses, and other healthcare practitioners address current ethical issues. These works cut through the usual back-and-forth of abstract arguments to examine how to resolve dilemmas in the clinic, at the bedside, and in the boardroom. Volumes address practical issues such as professionalism in healthcare, clinical bioethics consultation, death and dying, and clinical genetics. These books provide a distinctive resource for educating practitioners-in-training such as medical students and residents, allied health professionals, healthcare administrators, and policymakers, as well as students of bioethics at the graduate and undergraduate level.

Editorial Advisory Board

Titles in the Series

Death in the Clinic

Edited by Lynn A. Jansen

ROWMAN & LITTLEFIELD PUBLISHERS, INC.
Lanham • Boulder • New York • Toronto • Oxford

The poem "Do not go gentle into that good night," by Dylan Thomas, is reproduced in chapter 7 from Dylan Thomas, *The Poems of Dylan Thomas* (New York:
New Directions, 1952), 18. Copyright © 1952 by Dylan Thomas. Reprinted by
permission of New Directions Publishing Corp. The essay which makes up chapter
3 is reproduced with revision from J. David Velleman, "Against the Right to Die,"
The Journal of Medicine and Philosophy 17, no. 6 (1992): 665–81. Reprinted by
permission of Taylor & Francis, Inc. Permission to reprint this material is gratefully
acknowledged.

ROWMAN & LITTLEFIELD PUBLISHERS, INC.

Published in the United States of America
by Rowman & Littlefield Publishers, Inc.
A wholly owned subsidiary of The Rowman & Littlefield Publishing Group, Inc.
4501 Forbes Boulevard, Suite 200, Lanham, Maryland 20706
www.rowmanlittlefield.com

PO Box 317
Oxford
OX2 9RU, UK

Copyright © 2006 by Rowman & Littlefield Publishers, Inc.

British Library Cataloguing in Publication Information Available

Library of Congress Cataloging-in-Publication Data

Death in the clinic / edited by Lynn A. Jansen.
    p.   cm.— (Practicing bioethics)
   Includes bibliographical references and index.
   ISBN 0-7425-3509-6 (cloth : alk. paper)—ISBN 0-7425-3510-X
(pbk. : alk. paper)
    1. Terminal care—Moral and ethical aspects.   2. Death—Moral and ethical
aspects.   3. Death.
   [DNLM: 1. Terminal Care—ethics.   2. Attitude to Death.   3. Bioethical
Issues.   4. Terminally Ill—psychology. WB 310 D2844 2006]   I. Jansen, Lynn
A., 1963–
II. Series.
   R726.D442   2006
   179.7—dc22   2005025716

Printed in the United States of America

♾ ™ The paper used in this publication meets the minimum requirements of
American National Standard for Information Sciences—Permanence of Paper for
Printed Library Materials, ANSI/NISO Z39.48–1992.

Contents

v

Acknowledgments

I would like to express gratitude to Mark Kuczewski, the series editor of *Practicing Bioethics,* for asking me to edit this volume. Eve DeVaro and Tessa Fallon from Rowman & Littlefield provided helpful technical and administrative support. Finally, I would like to thank all of the contributors of this volume not only for agreeing to contribute their fine work to complete this project, but also for keeping their promises to do so according to schedule.

Introduction

Lynn A. Jansen

Over the past quarter century, a large and growing literature has been devoted to ethics at the end of life. Much of this literature engages with controversial issues that concern the termination of life and the discontinuation of medical interventions.[1] Topics like physician-assisted suicide and voluntary euthanasia not only have captured the public's mind, but also have dominated the academic discussion of end-of-life issues among clinicians, lawyers, and bioethicists. Surprisingly, however, little sustained attention has been paid to the topic of death itself and how thinking about death relates to and affects clinical practice.[2] This volume addresses a range of important ethical issues that clinicians confront in and around the fact that their patients die, as well as the ethical stance they should take toward the imminence (or occurrence) of the death of their patients.[3]

OLD PROBLEMS AND NEW CHALLENGES

Much of the early work on death and dying centered on the ethical problem of applying modern technology at the end of life. This concern tracked ongoing advances in medical technology and expressed the worry that patients were increasingly held hostage to the powers of technological development. Robert Veatch described the concern well:

Death, as never before, is looked upon as an evil, and we are mobilizing technology in an all-out war against it. If not death itself, at least certain types of
death are beginning to be seen as conquerable. We are being forced to ask the
question, "Is death moral in a technological age?"[4]

Quite understandably, then, this concern about technology in the clinic
motivated efforts to devise ethically defensible strategies for taming
what was seen to be a relentless therapeutic imperative to resist death.

Three assumptions informed these early efforts. The first assumption—*the privacy of death*—holds that individuals should be free to
"die on their own terms" and that death has a private meaning for each
person. The second assumption—*the centrality of autonomous
agency*—holds that individuals who are dying have the capacity (and
should be encouraged) to work out what death with dignity means to
them and to make use of legal instruments to ensure that their wishes
are respected. The third assumption—*the neutrality of clinical judgment*—holds that clinical judgment about the appropriate limits of medical interventions at the end of life should rest on general considerations
of medical/technological efficacy, rather than on quality of life judgments made by the individual physician.

These assumptions, and the ideas underlying them, defined a certain
approach to ethics at the end of life that has been dominant for the last
twenty-five years. They have also played a key role in the way clinicians
and clinical ethicists have been trained to think about and approach
death in the clinic. By now, most practicing clinicians are sensitive to
the moral value of looking for advance directives, incorporating the
patient's judgment into their medical decision making, and conceiving
the medical team more broadly to include more than the medical
experts at the bedside.

Yet despite success on these fronts, it has become increasingly clear
that more work needs to be done. A new approach to death and dying
is needed to complement the old. In 1997 the Institute of Medicine published a comprehensive assessment of the quality of care at the end of
life. This report made it plain that after nearly twenty-five years of ethical discussion addressing physician-assisted suicide, advance directives, and Do Not Resuscitate (DNR) orders, medical education still
does "not sufficiently prepare health professionals to recognize the final
phases of illness, understand and manage their own emotional reaction

to dying, construct effective strategies for care, and communicate sensitively to patients and those close to them."[5]

The chapters in this volume respond to this deficit in medical education by challenging the assumptions underlying early theorizing about death in the clinic. To see why it is necessary to challenge these assumptions, consider two problems that routinely confront clinicians who are concerned to help their patients die well. The first problem is that many of the patients who die in the modern hospital are not, at least not typically, ideal models of autonomous agency. Patients who die in the clinic are subject to various kinds of pressures and disabilities. Many are depressed, psychologically isolated, fearful, and in pain. Others lack decision-making capacity to various degrees and extents; and still others are financially burdened. All of these conditions can compromise the autonomous will of a dying patient.

This poses a problem for the clinician, since, on the assumption of the centrality of autonomous agency, the difficult issues concerning the value of prolonged life and the badness of death can (and should) be resolved by consulting the patient's will. But when the will of dying patients is compromised, then clinicians must take a much more active role in guiding patients and their families toward responsible medical decisions. This is made especially difficult by the fact that most dying patients do not have living wills or other advance directives.[6] Clinicians trained to depend on the centrality of autonomous agency for end of life decision making will be ill-equipped to help their patients in these contexts.

The second problem is that patients who die in the modern clinic often do not have stable, readily available support systems to guide them through the dying process in the clinical setting. Indeed, even when family members are present, there are often a number of factors, psychological and cultural, that make it difficult for them to participate in developing a plan of care for their loved one at the end of life. The fact of familial strain at the end of life poses a problem for clinicians trained to think of death as primarily a private matter, one in which patients in consultation with their family members decide how to die with dignity.

Taken together, these two problems illustrate how a reliance on a "traditional" end of life ethics curriculum alone can leave clinicians ill-prepared to construct effective and compassionate plans of care for their dying patients. The problems underscore the need to incorporate a new imperative into the old curriculum—one that encourages clinicians to reflect on the ethical significance of death and to develop a defensible ethical stance toward dying.

Yet if there is a need to reform medical education with respect to these matters, then how might this be accomplished? What can be done to help clinicians think more reflectively and compassionately about death and dying? Many have suggested that the best way to expose medical students and residents to death and dying is to introduce it to them through literature and clinical narratives.[7] Doing so makes medical education more humanistic. It has been less widely appreciated, however, that there is a role for theoretical or philosophical reflection on death and dying in medical education. Narrative can render the events surrounding death and dying in the clinic more intelligible. It can situate them within a story and thereby invest them with meaning. But while narrative can provide emotional understanding, it can also distort judgment.[8] People's attitudes toward dying are not always rational and their emotions toward the prospect of death are often unstable. If clinicians are to develop an ethically defensible stance toward death, then they will need to subject their own attitudes and emotions to critical scrutiny. It is here that theoretical reflection and philosophical analysis have a crucial role to play.

The chapters in this volume bring theoretical perspectives on death and the ethical issues that surround it into contact with a range of difficult problems that clinicians must deal with in the modern clinic. They look at some of the old problems through a new lens and seek to move beyond the important, but well-worn, discussion of the ethical limits of technology at the end of life. The chapters also bring into view, and critically examine, the meaning of clinicians' relationships to their dying or recently deceased patients and the various ways that a patient's death can destabilize the self-understanding of a clinician.

THEMES AND PERSPECTIVES

Several theoretical perspectives inform the chapters in this volume. Reviewing them will illuminate the importance, as well as the difficulty, of developing an ethically defensible stance toward death and incorporating it into medical practice. But first I enter a caveat. The authors in this volume do not agree on all matters. The chapters do not articulate a single, unified, shared ethical stance toward death. The theoretical perspectives surveyed below emerge from the volume as a whole.

The Public Meaning of Death

While death is a private event, it also has a public dimension. But what does this mean? For centuries philosophers have argued about the ethical significance of death. They have asked how death can be bad for the person who dies, and they have assumed that reasons and arguments can be given for different views on this question. They have assumed, in effect, that death has a public meaning—that it can be understood by rational methods of public argument.

In chapter 1, David Mayo addresses this aspect of the public meaning of death. In particular, Mayo explores the ethical relevance death has to the dying patient and to the health care provider who often forms a relationship with the patient. It is vital (but sometimes difficult) for clinicians not to run together the badness for them of the death of their patients with the badness of death for the patients who are dying.[9] Failure to keep these perspectives distinct can obscure the fact that life has a natural limit and it can encourage a tendency in physicians to overtreat their dying patients. Attention to the reasons why death is bad, and for whom it is bad, can help keep them from making this error.

The public meaning of death is not only evident in public reasoning about death and its significance, but also in controversies over when physicians should declare their patients dead. Plainly, if a patient has died, then medical interventions to keep the patient alive are pointless. But advances in medical technology have complicated the question of when patients die. The invention of the positive-pressure mechanical ventilator in the mid-twentieth century, for example, made it possible for profoundly brain-damaged patients to maintain cardiac and respiratory functions.[10] This raised the vexing question, is a patient with a complete and permanent loss of brain functions, who nonetheless continues to have a heartbeat, still alive?[11]

James Bernat provides a helpful survey of the main areas of public disagreement that fuel the controversy over defining death in chapter 2.

He then defends the whole-brain criterion of brain-death. While Bernat recognizes that this criterion for determining death in the clinic is still controversial,[12] he defends it because, in his view, it squares with our ordinary usage of the concept. Still, as Bernat would likely agree, the controversy over defining death is not merely a controversy over the correct analysis of a shared concept. It also expresses the deeper issue over the value of life and the badness of death.

This point becomes apparent when we reflect on the fact that the medical community must decide when it is appropriate to resist death and when it is appropriate to let patients die. There is a long tradition in medicine of limiting interventions in the face of approaching death. Distinctions—such as that between ordinary and extraordinary treatment and proportionate and disproportionate burdens and benefits—have been formulated to help clinicians think about this matter. These distinctions, however, rest ultimately on judgments about the value of mortal life. They pull us beyond the scientific authority of medicine and into the evaluative domain, a domain that is much broader than medicine. The problem of limiting medical interventions to prolong life must rest in the end on a public consensus about the value of human life.

The need to reach a public consensus on this matter, as John Paris, Michael D. Schreiber, and Robert Fogerty point out in chapter 7, shows that the problem of developing an ethically defensible stance toward death is not merely a problem for clinicians, but one for the wider society as well. Individual clinicians and medical societies, however, can play an important role in helping to shape this consensus. By formulating clear clinical standards for limiting medical interventions and outlining the ethical rationales for these limits, they can contribute to the public task of reaching a reasoned consensus on when it is right to let patients die.[13]

Traditional end of life ethics places heavy emphasis on the limits of medicine. But the acceptance of these limits does not bring with it a genuine understanding of the ways in which death can be a positive good (or bad) for one's self (as a clinician and a person) and for one's patient. Nor does it bring with it an understanding of how to manage the destabilizing effects of death. These issues require public, ethical reasoning for their resolution, but they are largely ignored in contemporary medical education.

Patient Autonomy and Clinical Neutrality

The task of developing an ethically defensible stance toward death is, as I noted above, complicated by the fact that dying patients are often not fully autonomous agents. The centrality of patient autonomy in modern clinical ethics has, at least in some respects, made it easier for clinicians to avoid confronting the hard questions about death and dying. Without question, respect for patient autonomy is necessary to ensure proper respect for the individual patient. This is one of the central truths of modern medical ethics. But the expectation that dying patients will in fact be fully competent to participate in medical decision making at the end of life has brought with it a largely unexamined ethical stance toward death.

Clinicians, it is frequently said, must not impose their own ethical views on their dying patients. To respect the autonomy of their patients, they must present them with the full range of available medical options and then remain neutral on the ethical value of these options. Medical students, in particular, commonly fall back on this stance when asked to reason about medical ethics for the first time. They adopt a posture of neutrality, one that (seemingly) avoids imposing *their* ethical views on their patients.

Yet, as several chapters in this volume bring out, the relationship between respect for patient autonomy at the end of life and clinical neutrality is far from straightforward. J. David Velleman explores some of the complexities that surround this issue in a penetrating discussion of the institutional "right to die" in chapter 3. Velleman rejects this right on the grounds that it can make dying patients worse off. When a dying patient is given the option to terminate his life, he becomes responsible for exercising or failing to exercise that option. The patient now must justify his decision *not* to exercise the option, and this can be a burden that he would be better off not having.

Velleman's discussion nicely brings into view the pressures, both financial and emotional, that can impinge on the decision making of an elderly or terminally ill patient. Paradoxically (although Velleman does not put the point exactly this way), by increasing the choices of dying patients, we can decrease their autonomy by putting them in situations where they feel pressured to make choices that they wish they did not have to make.

If Velleman is right, then clinicians cannot avoid difficult ethical decisions simply by presenting their patients with a full range of medical options and then deferring to their judgment. There is a prior issue about which medical options should be presented to dying patients, and this issue presents questions that pull one beyond the posture of clinical neutrality. Indeed, merely informing a patient that he or she has a certain option, such as the option voluntarily to refuse food and fluids to precipitate death, can, at least in some circumstances, make the physician complicit in the patient's decision to exercise that option.[14]

Respect for autonomy and clinical neutrality can come apart in a more direct way as well. Patients who die in the modern clinic, as I have stressed, often suffer from conditions that impair to varying degrees the cognitive abilities necessary for autonomous agency as well as the capacities needed to make voluntary decisions. Those who treat dying patients, therefore, frequently confront the task of determining when a patient has and does not have the capacity to make his or her own medical decisions.

What values should guide clinicians in making this assessment? Linda Ganzini and Elizabeth Goy in chapter 5 point out that, given the difficulties of making clinical assessments of decision-making competence at the end of life, we should not be surprised to find that these assessments are often informed by ethical as well as clinical considerations. They point to a study of standards for competence to pursue physician-assisted suicide showing that forensic psychiatrists who were morally opposed to this practice were more likely to advocate more stringent standards for competence assessment than those who did not have moral objections to the practice.

The results of this study suggest that clinical and ethical judgments are often intertwined in ways that may not be fully transparent to the practicing clinician. Despite the emphasis on clinical neutrality in modern medical ethics, unexamined assumptions about the value of life and death often inform clinical practice. The remedy for this problem is not to tell clinicians to try harder to be neutral, however. Clinicians who treat dying patients need to become aware of, and be willing to subject to critical scrutiny, the ethical assumptions that inform their practice. This, it should be stressed, is not an invitation for them to impose their own idiosyncratic views on their patients. It is rather an invitation for clinicians to participate with others in the medical profession in developing a publicly defensible ethical stance toward death and dying.

Respect and Cultural Norms

I have been discussing the public meaning of death and the need for public reasoning concerning the stance clinicians should take toward their dying patients. But any adequate account of these matters must be sensitive to the multicultural context of the modern hospital. Death is an event with great social and religious significance. Differing cultural attitudes toward death affect what counts as respectful treatment of dying, and recently deceased, patients. This brings us to a third theoretical perspective that is explored in this volume.

Respect for persons is a universal norm, but its application is sensitive to cultural difference. Those who treat dying patients need to know more than what is provided by the medical history and physical examinations of their patients. They also need to inquire into the social circumstances and cultural beliefs of those they treat. Only by doing so can they provide optimal care to their patients while respecting them as "whole persons."

In chapter 6, Celia Berdes and Linda Emanuel explore this idea in the specific context of geriatric medicine. They discuss the importance of "comprehensive assessment" in treating the elderly and the dying. Comprehensive assessment is based on the idea that without a full understanding of the patient, it is not possible to develop an optimal plan of care for him or her. As Berdes and Emanuel point out, patients and their families often do not have a clear understanding of their own goals for care.

Comprehensive assessment is particularly important for those who are very old or terminally ill. Old age and serious illness bring special and difficult challenges—such as the loss of independence, the progressive loss of mental and physical functioning, and the loss of a secure sense of self. To respond well to these challenges, patients need to develop the ability to adapt to them; and this requires those who care for them to attend to their cultural beliefs and social needs.

The relationship between the norm of respect for persons and its relation to social and cultural difference is also illuminatingly explored by Mark Wicclair in chapter 8, which also discusses the practice of using newly deceased patients for purposes of medical training. After discussing the advantages of using dead humans to train medical students, Wicclair asks whether the practice is ethically defensible. He argues that the practice is not *per se* unethical, but that it can become unethical if it uses the deceased person in a way that he or she would have considered disrespectful.

The respectful treatment of corpses varies considerably between cultures. One reason for this is that different religions and social groups view the connection between a person and a person's body after death in very different ways. Given these differences, it is important to inquire into the wishes of the deceased patient and his or her family. At the minimum, respecting the bodies of deceased patients requires honoring their premortem decisions (if any were made) or complying with their premortem preferences (if any are known). Absent evidence of premortem decisions or preferences, Wicclair concludes that using the body of a newly deceased patient for medical training is not ethically permissible unless his or her family has given their consent.

THE CLINICAL CONTEXT

The theoretical issues reviewed above are encountered by clinicians in the institutional context of the modern hospital. There are a variety of factors, cultural and legal, that help define this context; and these factors contribute to the difficulty of developing an ethically defensible approach to the treatment of dying patients. For this reason, any realistic discussion of death and dying in the clinic requires that the institutional setting of the modern hospital be kept in view.

The rise of the palliative care movement is a case in point. Over the past twenty-five years, palliative care medicine has made great progress in helping dying patients and their families achieve the best possible quality of life. Countless patients have been helped to achieve a more comfortable death as a result of palliative care measures. Still, as David Barnard points out in chapter 4, the clinical success of palliative care medicine must be celebrated with a measure of caution. This success has contributed to the emergence of a set of attitudes among end of life practitioners that Barnard terms "palliative care triumphalism." This is the "tendency to equate palliative medicine's growing sophistication in symptom management, and in the orchestration of the dying process according to various pharmacological, psychological, and social protocols, with the mastery of the problem of death."[15]

The danger of palliative care triumphalism is that it can become yet another way for clinicians to avoid dealing with the reality and imminence of their patients' death. As Barnard puts it, palliative medicine goes wrong "when our proliferating techniques for easing the process of dying are confused with a means to protect patients and carers from the de-centering, disruptive power of death."[16] Viewed in this way, palliative care triumphalism runs the risk of becoming just a new instantiation of the attempt to control death by technological means.

A second factor that conditions the institutional reality of death in the clinic is one that I have stressed throughout this introduction. Patients who are able to communicate their wishes, fears, and concerns about their own death are patients who can participate in the kind of relationship that is so valued in palliative care. But, sadly, many patients at the end of life are unable to engage in these relationships. According to the Institute of Medicine, more than 70 percent of those who die each year are elderly.[17] Many of these patients will die because of, or while suffering from, advanced dementia. Other patients will die suffering from varying degrees of depression or more severe forms of mental illness, such as schizophrenia. Little research has been done to understand how these groups of patients experience death and the dying process. Nor has much attention been paid to what level of palliative care patients with severe mental illnesses, like schizophrenia, receive, if any.[18]

A final institutional feature of the modern clinic should be mentioned. Much of this volume focuses on the role of theoretical reflection in helping clinicians to develop an ethically defensible stance toward death in the clinic. However, as I have alluded to, this is generally not something each physician is free to do alone, in isolation. The attitudes that clinicians have toward death in general and the reactions that they have to the dying of their own patients in particular take place within a background of social and legal framework. Law, public policy, and regulatory bodies have enormous influence on how clinicians react to the dying of their patients. As several of the writers in this volume make plain, judicial and legal actions over the past thirty years have not only shaped how the medical community defines death, but also clarified the ways in which physicians may help their terminally ill patients through the dying process.

There is, however, always a potential tension between the requirements of law and ethics. The fear of legal reprisals or sanctions may lead some physicians to avoid doing all they can to relieve the pain and suffering of their dying patients. Similarly, concern about malpractice litigation may lead others to practice defensive medicine on their terminally ill patients and, thereby, unnecessarily extend their lives and worsen their deaths.[19] The chapters in this volume discuss some of these tensions between law and ethics.

CONCLUSION

Death in the Clinic fills a gap in contemporary medical education. It takes seriously the Institute of Medicine's recommendation that clinicians and educators should be encouraged to acknowledge and incorporate into their curriculum "the reality that people die and that dying patients are not people for whom 'nothing can be done.'"[20]

The volume aims primarily to provide medical students, residents, and medical educators a framework within which they might begin to explore and deal with this reality. But, as I have stressed, working out an ethically defensible stance toward death is not a task that belongs solely to physicians. While medical students and medical residents will find the issues raised in this book particularly relevant, the focus on existential and philosophical questions about death should also make the book of interest to chaplains, social workers, palliative care clinicians, nurses, and clinical ethicists.

Death in the Clinic does not provide a full treatment of all issues surrounding the ethics of death and dying. The range of issues covered here is intended to bring readers into contact with some of the concrete ethical issues that concern death and dying that arise on a daily basis in the clinical setting. These are issues that clinicians, patients, and their families continue to struggle with, despite the best efforts of medical ethicists over the past quarter century to resolve them. *Death in the Clinic* does not offer the last word on any of the theoretical issues about the nature of death that it raises. Developing an ethically defensible stance toward death is a daunting task. It begins with a clear recognition of the problem and its difficulty. My hope is that this volume will assist clinicians in taking this important first step.

NOTES

1. See, for example, Tom L. Beauchamp and Seymour Perlin, *Ethical Issues in Death and Dying* (Englewood, N.J.: Prentice Hall, 1978); Robert M. Veatch, *Death, Dying and the Biological Revolution: Our Last Quest for Responsibility* (New Haven, Conn.: Yale University Press, 1976); and M. P. Battin, R. Rhodes, and A. Silvers, *Physician Assisted Suicide: Expanding the Debate* (New York: Routledge, 1998).

2. But see Daniel Callahan, "Pursuing a Peaceful Death," *The Hastings Center Report* 23 (July–August 1993): 33–38; and William Joseph Gavin, *Cuttin' the Body Loose: Historical, Biological, and Personal Approaches to Death and Dying* (Philadelphia: Temple University Press, 1995).

3. A number of topics are not discussed in this book. These include double effect, doing and allowing, terminal sedation, etc. There are a number of excellent books that address these topics. Interested readers should consult, for example, Battin, Rhodes, and Silvers, *Physician Assisted Suicide*.

4. Robert M. Veatch, *Death, Dying and the Biological Revolution: Our Last Quest for Responsibility* (New Haven, Conn.: Yale University Press, 1976), 3.

5. Mary J. Field and Christine K. Cassell, eds., *Approaching Death: Improving Care at the End of Life* (Washington, D.C.: National Academy Press, 1997), 6.

6. Field and Cassell, eds., *Approaching Death*, 202–3.

7. See for example, Timothy E. Quill, *A Midwife Through the Dying Process: Stories of Healing and Hard Choices at the End of Life* (Baltimore, Md.: Johns Hopkins University Press, 1996); I. Byock, *Dying Well: The Prospect of Growth at the End of Life* (New York: Riverhead, 1997); and David Barnard et al., *Crossing Over: Narratives of Palliative Care* (Oxford: Oxford University Press, 2000). See also Field and Cassell, eds., *Approaching Death*, 218.

8. See, for example, the discussion of the "projective error" in J. David Velleman, "Narrative Explanation," *Philosophical Review* 112, no. 1 (2003): 1–25.

9. David J. Mayo, "Some Reflections on Whether Death Is Bad," in *Death in the Clinic*, ed. Lynn A. Jansen (Lanham, Md.: Rowman & Littlefield, 2006).

10. James L. Bernat, "Defining Death," in *Death in the Clinic*, ed. Lynn A. Jansen (Lanham, Md.: Rowman & Littlefield, 2006).

11. Bernat, "Defining Death."

12. See, for example, Robert Veatch, "The Impending Collapse of the Whole–Brain Definition of Death," *Hastings Center Report* (July–August 1993): 18–24.

13. John J. Paris, Michael D. Schreiber, and Robert Fogerty, "Rage, Rage

against the Dying of the Light: Not a Metaphor for End-of-Life Care," in *Death in the Clinic*, ed. Lynn A. Jansen (Lanham, Md.: Rowman & Littlefield, 2006).

14. Lynn A. Jansen, "No Safe Harbor: The Principle of Complicity and the Practice of Voluntary Stopping of Eating and Drinking," *The Journal of Medicine and Philosophy* 29 (February 2004): 61–75.

15. David Barnard, "The Skull at the Banquet," in *Death in the Clinic*, ed. Lynn A. Jansen (Lanham, Md.: Rowman & Littlefield, 2006).

16. Barnard, "The Skull at the Banquet."

17. Field and Cassell, eds., *Approaching Death*, 2.

18. Linda Ganzini and Elizabeth R. Goy, "Influence of Mental Illness on Decision Making at the End of Life," in *Death in the Clinic*, ed. Lynn A. Jansen (Lanham, Md.: Rowman & Littlefield, 2006).

19. Field and Cassell, eds., *Approaching Death*.

20. Field and Cassell, eds., *Approaching Death*, 9.

1

THE PUBLIC MEANING OF DEATH

1

Some Reflections on Whether Death Is Bad

David J. Mayo

Is death bad? It certainly seems so to most people. All of us are saddened at the deaths of those who are close to us, and we ordinarily do not look forward to our own deaths. But death is perfectly natural by any definition of the term. Why exactly, then, is it bad, for whom is it bad, and wherein does its badness consist?

I begin to explore these questions in part I with a short summary of reasons that a person's death is typically bad for survivors. I then turn in part II to the more difficult and elusive question of whether a person's death is bad for that person. In part III, I relate these philosophical reflections to the clinical context. Health care providers who treat patients with terminal illnesses must deal with death on a regular basis. But medical education standardly does not train physicians to think about the significance of death. A more reflective understanding of the badness of death can enable them to approach the death of their patients with an appropriate attitude. This, in turn, may lead them to provide better care to their dying patients.

THE BADNESS OF DEATH FOR SURVIVORS

The misfortune someone's death represents for survivors is relatively straightforward. We are above all social creatures. Our own welfare is

17

intimately bound up, in various ways, with that of those around us. Others are often key players in many of the projects that give our lives meaning. The sudden death of a thesis advisor or business partner, for example, could be a loss that seriously interrupts one's career or business. Loved ones, in particular, tend to figure in our most central projects (e.g., raising children, sharing our lives with close friends and spouses). Their deaths bring these valuable projects to an end. Moreover, true friendship and love involve wanting to see the friend or beloved flourish, quite apart from any role we may play in that flourishing. Their good fortune is our good fortune, and their misfortune ours, simply because we care about them. If their flourishing is cut short, we suffer the loss of the good that their flourishing would have represented to them and hence to us.

Moreover, the loss of a loved one often has a fallout effect beyond the immediate circle. Because I care about my friend, I am saddened by his sorrow at the death of his mother, in spite of having never met her (just as I am saddened by his sorrow at the death of his dog, in spite of having disliked the dog). To the extent that we feel a general sympathy for our fellow creatures, we are saddened even to hear of the deaths of strangers, knowing they leave behind grieving parents, children, husbands, or wives whose lives will now be the poorer.

In all of these ways, then, the death of a person can easily be bad for others. The badness or misfortune can consist first in the cutting short of projects that we value and give our lives meaning, and second in the feelings of pain and sadness that accompany the realization that these losses have been suffered by ourselves, or by others for whom we feel sympathy.

THE BADNESS OF DEATH FOR THE PERSON WHOSE DEATH IS AT ISSUE

Philosophically, the question of whether a person's death is bad for the deceased person is much more perplexing. We often presume it is so. Again, people ordinarily do not look forward to their own death, and some are terrified by the prospect of it. In addition, the experience of grief felt by survivors at the loss of loved ones seems to involve more than just *their* loss: it seems to focus as well on the apparent misfortune of the deceased.

Philosophers have wondered, is this judgment defensible? Is death really bad for the deceased? Epicurus and Thomas Nagel are two philosophers whose arguments regarding this question deserve our consideration.

Epicurus

In "A Letter to Menoeceus," Epicurus, a third-century B.C. Greek atomist, argues for the startling conclusion that death is not bad, and we are foolish to worry about it. He believed this followed from two key tenets of his worldview. First, he espoused hedonism, the view that in the final analysis only pleasure and pain are good and bad. Second, as an atomist he believed consciousness ends at death. He concluded that death should be of no concern for the wise person: death is neither pleasant nor painful, and hence neither good nor bad.

Epicurus supported this claim with several auxiliary arguments: since we ourselves each end at death, literally speaking there will be no time at which any of us will exist but be dead. Moreover, it is foolish to fear what will not be bad when it happens, so it is foolish to fear one's own death.

> Become accustomed to the belief that death is nothing to us. For all good and evil consists in sensation, but death is privation of sensation. And therefore a right understanding that death is nothing to us makes the mortality of life enjoyable, not because it adds to it an infinite span of time, but because it takes away the craving for immortality. . . . [T]he man speaks but idly who says that he fears death not because it will be painful when it comes, but because it is painful in anticipation. For that which gives no trouble when it comes, is but an empty pain in anticipation. So death, the most terrifying of ills, is nothing to us, since so long as we exist, death is not with us, but when death comes, then we do not exist. It does not then concern either the living or the dead, since for the former it is not, and the latter are no more.[1]

What can we say about Epicurus's claims? First, at best, Epicurus has only shown that being dead is not bad. This does not preclude the very real possibility of dying being bad by virtue of being painful. Moreover, it only speaks in part to the grief survivors feel upon the death of a loved one. Even if Epicurus is right that we should not grieve for the deceased (as I believe most of us are often inclined to do), his argument says nothing about the pain we feel over the loss their death represents in our own lives, or in the lives of other survivors.

Notwithstanding these qualifications, Epicurus's argument still stands at odds with the widespread conviction that the prospect of death is the prospect of a very real misfortune and hence that fearing it is not foolish. Is this intuition mistaken, or is Epicurus's argument specious?

I share Epicurus's conviction that consciousness ends at death: the evidence that it depends on some level of brain function strikes me as overpowering. I will simply assume that point in what follows, and not argue it, not because I assume all readers will agree, but because further argument on that point would take us too far afield. For those who believe in some form of afterlife, it seems clear that their view of the afterlife will be determinative of their view of the (positive or negative) value of death.

But what of Epicurus's claim "all good and evil consists in sensation"? Here the situation is somewhat more complicated. I believe Epicurus is right that ultimately what makes a life valuable derives from the value of the experiences it does, or might, contain. I doubt many people who value their life would be anxious to extend it by fifty years of irreversible coma. However I have reservations about Epicurus's simple hedonism. An experience might be rich and valued without being "pleasant," e.g., the experience of giving birth, or of arriving in time to be present at the death of a parent.

Still, if experience ends at death, and if all value is somehow rooted in experience, is Epicurus right that all value ends at death? I believe he is not, for reasons clearly laid out by a contemporary philosopher, Thomas Nagel.

Thomas Nagel

Nagel[2] shares with Epicurus and myself the conviction that consciousness ends at death and hence that being dead will not be painful. He argues, however, that death can be bad as the deprivation of goods that further life might have offered. Nagel's fundamental dispute with Epicurus is over his conviction that the deprivation of a good can itself amount to a genuine misfortune. Thus even if the origin of value is ultimately to be found in certain valued experiences, the deprivation of good experiences may be legitimately viewed as bad or unfortunate. The baseball fan holding tickets to a World Series game suffers a genuine misfortune if he gets caught in heavy traffic and misses the game.

At first glance it might seem (in keeping with the spirit of Epicurus's argument that all value lies in *actual* experiences) that the misfortune here is grounded in the anguish he experiences while caught in the traffic. (It is not difficult to picture the frantic fan, looking alternately at his watch and the stationary traffic ahead of him.) Against this Nagel argues, rightly in my view, that even deprivations of which one is not aware may be genuine misfortunes. Imagine I mail two tickets to a 2004 World Series game to a friend who is a Red Sox fan as a surprise birthday present. Imagine in addition they get lost in the mail. Nagel's point is that my friend suffers a misfortune even if he never learns of it. (Indeed Nagel would argue a misfortune has occurred even if neither of us ever realized what happened.) Of course, if I later learn of the misfortune from a third party, I would be well advised not to tell my friend, for this would upset him. But the reason he would be upset (and the reason our friend in traffic was upset) was because he knew of the misfortune he was suffering. (Why else would he be upset?) It only makes sense to be upset about bad things. Unless missing the game itself was a misfortune, it would be foolish to be upset about it.

While I am sympathetic to Nagel's conviction that the deprivation of a good can be a misfortune, and hence that death can be bad as the deprivation of the goods one's life would have contained had one not died, this view is not without its problems. In particular, if we accept it, how bad someone's death is for them will depend on what goods their life would have contained had death not intervened. Some deaths strike us as more tragic than others in just this way. Intuitively, for instance, death at 20 is worse than death at 90, and Nagel's "deprivation" account lends itself to an obvious explanation of why this is so. But how are we to generalize this account? Since the goods of which death deprives us never happen, how in general is one to make sense of what goods those would have been? It's easy enough to gauge how bad it is to have my one-hour massage abruptly cut short by twenty minutes, because we have a pretty clear idea of how things would almost certainly have unfolded but for the cutting short. With death, however, it is difficult to attach precise content to this counterfactual notion of how things might have played out but for the death. Nagel grants this is a sticking point in his analysis. He considers the option of appealing to a "normal life span," but rejects this approach, in spite of the fact that it accounts for the view that a "premature" death is worse than a death at 90, because he feels it will strike the 90-year-old as un-compelling. While "observed from without" death at 90 may seem natural enough, "the trouble is that life familiarizes us with the goods of which death deprives us,"[3] and "a man's sense of his own experience does not embody this idea of a natural limit." Nagel's idea seems to be that living life is typically *not* like eating a meal, where the pleasures of eating slowly diminish as one approaches satiety. "[Man] finds himself the subject of a *life*, with an indeterminate and not essentially limited future. Viewed in this way, death, no matter how inevitable, is an abrupt cancellation of indefinitely extensive possible goods." Nagel concludes ". . . it may be that a bad end is in store for us all."[4]

Against Nagel's analysis here, I wish to advance the following two considerations. First, it strikes me that Nagel is simply wrong when he suggests that everyone ("as the subject of a life") views his or her future as "indeterminate and not essentially limited," and hence that death is viewed by every subject as "an abrupt cancellation of indefinitely extensive possible goods." This may be true of some people—those who have never really "come to terms with death"—young people who feel they are invincible, for instance, or those who have always enjoyed good health and are not given to pondering "the big questions." One can even imagine the extremely vigorous—and optimistic—ninety-year-old who envisions her future as something as open-ended as Nagel describes. But this may not be a rational attitude to take toward one's own future. Certainly, many people see their futures otherwise. Let me suggest some possibilities.

Far from taking their future for granted, some people who have had "a close brush with death" are very much aware that their life is finite, regard each day as even more precious for that reason, and try to live each day to the fullest and revel in the goods it contains. Still others begin to grow weary of their lives as they age, finding less and less joy to outweigh the mounting losses that typically accompany progressive degenerative diseases and the aging process. Again, friendships with loved ones figure prominently among the goods most of us value most highly, and for the very elderly these goods diminish as loved ones are lost to death. Many people facing incapacitating critical—and potentially fatal—illness would actually prefer death to further life involving life-prolonging therapies which at best may offer only a marginal prolongation of a painful existence. Further, they understand that medicine can only postpone death, not eliminate it. The new medical technologies that make possible the prolongation of life are sometimes unwelcome. Thus end-of-life care is no longer governed by the paternalistic Vitalist imperative to prolong life whenever possible, but rather by the doctrine of informed consent, and the right of patients to determine, perhaps by a written advance directive, whether to forgo even life-sustaining therapy when things get to a certain point of diminishing returns.

These are certainly not "happy" situations. However, I suggest that what is bad in many of them is not death, but the inevitable losses of age and disease which diminish the goods of life, while adding to its sorrows. In such cases death itself can be a positive good.

There is a second point on which I take issue with Nagel: while I agree that the deprivation of a good can be a misfortune, I believe the good in question must be one that is probable or likely, not merely one that is conceivable. Moreover, the less likely it is, the less its deprivation should be considered a genuine misfortune. Not winning the lottery or being the richest person on earth are not misfortunes, and if someone experiences disappointment on either of these counts, the fundamental misfortune is that the person should have held the unrealistic expectations which give rise to the disappointment. (A friend and I have a running joke; whenever a minor misfortune, e.g. misplaced keys, besets either of us, he cries "First I lose the lottery, and now this!!!")

We are brought, then, to the following general conclusions about the badness of death. We must distinguish between the perspective of the deceased and that of survivors. Regarding the former, I have suggested the most defensible view is to be found between Nagel and Epicurus: a "premature" death is bad to the extent it represents the loss of life-goods one might reasonably have expected. But for many people who are very elderly or critically ill, there simply is no longer any such reasonable expectation. Indeed, for those who die by their own decision in refusing further life-prolonging therapies (and perhaps with hospice care) death may be genuinely welcome—a genuine good. Thus we often

say and hear—admittedly at a time when we are more concerned with
comforting than with precision—"her death was a blessing." Regarding the latter, someone's death can be bad for survivors in two different
ways: first, lives are upset when key players in those lives are no longer
there to participate. In particular, loving survivors will almost inevitably suffer the painful personal loss of the love and friendship of the
deceased. Moreover, if the person's death is a misfortune for the
deceased, it will also be bad for those who love and care enough about
them to share in their misfortunes, as well as for those who love and
care about those who are grieving.

CLINICAL IMPLICATIONS

The foregoing discussion has implications for clinical practice. Clinicians who provide care to dying patients confront the issue of the badness of death from both of the perspectives discussed above, that of the
survivor and that of the person who dies. Clinicians form relationships
with their patients. Just as the death of a friend or colleague can be bad
for us, the death of a patient can be bad for the health care provider. It
is also possible that a physician may view his or her patient as a professional project. The physician may view the death of the patient as the
failure of his project to keep the patient alive and healthy. In addition,
clinicians confront the issue of the badness of death from the perspective of their patients. They can ask whether their dying patients will be
deprived of the kind of goods that would make death a misfortune.

In practice, and in the absence of theoretical reflection, it may be difficult for clinicians to distinguish these two perspectives on the badness
of death. They may run together the badness *for them* of the death of
their patient with the badness of death for the patient who is deceased.
But, as we have seen, the two perspectives present different concerns.
How then should a clinician think about the death of his dying patients?

It seems natural to think that the clinician's primary concern should
be with the perspective of the dying patient. His or her attitude toward
the patient's death should be informed by a judgment about whether or
not death would be bad for the patient. With this in mind, the clinician
should recognize that we are all subject to disease and, if we live long
enough, general infirmity and decline. These basic facts directly relate

to our earlier discussion of the badness of death. The death of a patient with an incapacitating and painful critical illness may not be a misfortune. It may even be a positive good for the patient. Likewise, if we believe that life has a natural limit—that is, if we reject Nagel's view of our future as open-ended and unlimited—then we may realize that the death of a very elderly patient would not be bad for the patient, for it may not bring with it the loss of reasonably expected goods.

Recognizing these points can enable clinicians to develop a more rational attitude toward the death of their dying patients. It also can help them to come to a better understanding of their own clinical practice and its limits. Health care providers who inevitably view the death of any patient as a medical or personal failure have set the bar for their own success unreasonably high. Their role is not to do what cannot be done, but only to do what is within their power to enhance the quality of the life of their patients.

This is no small matter. There are serious costs, for both health care providers and for patients, for setting the bar unreasonably high in this way. It will be costly for health care providers because the appropriate sadness they experience at the loss of a patient they have cared for and cared about will be irrationally amplified by the judgment of personal and professional failure.

More importantly, viewing death in the clinic as always a failure will be costly for patients. This is true for several reasons. First, it will encourage the "technological imperative" to overtreat. For centuries health care was guided by Medical Vitalism, the view that Death is the enemy, and that the physician's role is always to do whatever possible to preserve human life. This made good sense at a time when people tended to die, often quite young, of sudden-onset infections and other conditions, which could strike and cut life short quite suddenly. Today, however, people tend to die more slowly, and of chronic, degenerative conditions such as heart disease or other major organ failure, cancer, diabetes, or Alzheimer's. In many of these situations medicine can prolong life (and dying) beyond the point where further life rationally can be viewed as a benefit. Of course it would be best if such patients could be restored to a quality of life they valued. (It would be better for me if I won the lottery.) But where that is simply not possible—or where the patient simply doesn't want to assume the burdens involved in the gamble that it might be possible, patients suffer if the health care worker's tendency to view any patient's death as a failure results in overtreatment.

A CONCLUDING THOUGHT

There is a final and somewhat more speculative implication of our analysis. While some health care providers may assume patients inevitably look to them for a cure, what dying patients may want most of all—particularly if they accept the fact that their life is coming to a close—is the assurance that they will not be abandoned by their primary caregivers. Those who provide care to hospice patients, in a context where both patient and caregivers understand death is inevitable and that health care in this context consists above all in caring, do not find this depressing work. On the contrary, many of them tend to speak of how richly rewarding it can be to comfort the dying. One reason most dying patients never see their physicians once they enter a home hospice program is that physicians no longer make house calls. I wonder if perhaps physicians aren't themselves being shortchanged here. Quite apart from the question of what value physician visits might have for hospice patients, mightn't they help dispel any tendency of the physician to presume that a patient's death is always bad?

NOTES

1. Epicurus, "Letter to Menoeceus," *Epicurus: The Extant Remains*, trans. Cyril Bailey (Oxford: Clarendon Press, 1926), 85.

2. Thomas Nagel, "Death," in *Mortal Questions* (Cambridge: Cambridge University Press, 1979).

3. Nagel, "Death," 9–10.

4. Nagel, "Death," 10.

2

Defining Death

James L. Bernat

> The boundaries which divide Life from Death are, at best, shadowy and vague. Who shall say where the one ends, and where the other begins?
>
> —Edgar Allen Poe, *The Premature Burial*, 1844

Defining death is one of the oldest and most enduring problems in medicine, bioethics, and biophilosophy. Solving this problem was one of the first projects of the newly formed Institute of Society, Ethics, and the Life Sciences, later known as the Hastings Center.[1] It was also the first project of the President's Commission for the Study of Ethical Problems in Medicine and Biomedical and Behavioral Research.[2] Today, the problem of defining death continues to be debated in scholarly articles and books. What accounts for its fascination and staying power?

A MODERN HISTORY OF DEATH

Since the eighteenth century, physicians and scholars have debated important questions about death, such as whether the absence of heartbeat and breathing are death itself or merely indicators that death has occurred.[3] From the mid-eighteenth century through the end of the nineteenth century, physicians developed elaborate tests for death to attempt to eliminate incorrect determinations.[4] These physicians recognized the mutual interdependence of the vital systems of life: breathing, heartbeat-circulation, and brain functions. When one vital system ceased, the others ceased immediately because of their interdependence. Because bodily disintegration rapidly and inevitably followed the loss of these vital functions, these physicians could use the determination of the cessation of vital functions as highly accurate signs of death. Consequently, the permanent loss of vital functions became for some time the indisputable standard of death.

Mid-twentieth-century advances in medical technology, however, forever complicated the earlier straightforward determination of death. These advances permitted a dissociation of what had been mutually interdependent vital functions. The invention of the positive-pressure mechanical ventilator in the mid-twentieth century allowed a profoundly brain-damaged patient's respiration (that formerly would have ceased) to be maintained mechanically and, consequentially, her heartbeat and circulation could be supported, despite her complete and permanent loss of brain functions.

Now it could be asked, was such a patient alive or dead? The patient had some features traditionally associated with life, namely continued heartbeat, circulation of blood, air exchange in the lungs, digestion, and excretion. But she also had some features traditionally seen in death, such as the complete absence of brain functions, utter lack of movement and reflex responses, and an absence of breathing when the ventilator was disconnected. Based upon the traditional concept of death that requires interdependence of vital systems, the determination of whether the patient was alive or dead now was ambiguous because it was unclear which systems were essential for life. Although the advances in technology had not changed the concept of death, they made us aware that we had never previously discerned an explicit definition of death. That task had been unnecessary in the pretechnologic era when a dissociation of vital systems was impossible.[5]

The positive-pressure ventilator enabled patients who had suffered complete brain destruction to maintain, at least temporarily, heartbeat and circulation. These patients exhibited a depth of coma and loss of neurological functions that were so profound and different from previously described cases that French neurologists labeled them *le coma dépasseé* (a state beyond coma).[6] Increasingly, scholars began to claim that such patients were in fact dead, despite their retained heartbeat and circulation. In 1968 the Harvard Medical School Ad Hoc Committee

Report advanced a highly publicized and influential version of this claim.[7] It asserted that patients who had permanently lost all brain functions were dead.

The committee's report also popularized the unfortunate term "brain death." This term referred to the idea that a human with complete and irreversible cessation of brain functions was dead irrespective of continued mechanically maintained ventilation and circulation. However, the term "brain death" is a misleading and unfortunate term, since it wrongly implies that only the brain is dead and that there is more than one type of death. Nonetheless, the term resonated with the public and academy and has remained firmly entrenched in common usage.

Over the next several decades, the concept of brain death gained widespread acceptance and now is used by physicians in at least eighty countries.[8] The concept is supported in statute or administrative regulation in every state in the United States[9] and in all Canadian provinces. It is practiced throughout the Western world, and in many parts of the non-Western world including Islamic, Hindi, and Confucian-Buddhist cultures.[10] Some influential bioethicists have claimed that the enactment of more-or-less uniform laws governing brain death constitute evidence that the formerly contentious question of when a person is dead has now been resolved.[11]

Yet, within scholarly circles, debate on the definition of death continues to rage. Scholarly articles continue to be published claiming that brain death is conceptually incoherent,[12] a legal fiction,[13] and an anachronism that should be abandoned.[14] It is ironic that the largest number of critical scholarly articles and conferences on brain death has appeared during the very decade that has witnessed its greatest worldwide acceptance.[15] In this chapter, I have two objectives: first, to review the basis for the ongoing debate on defining death by identifying the remaining areas of disagreement; and, second, to defend a definition embracing whole-brain death.

WHY DEFINING DEATH IS IMPORTANT

A few scholars have argued that defining death is an unimportant and irrelevant task so long as society can agree on a set of rules for declaring death and for conducting social practices related to death, such as organ transplantation.[16] For example, Norman Fost maintains that the social purposes for declaring a patient dead (e.g., cessation of treatment, organ removal, settling estates, and burial) do not require a settled definition of death. Each of these purposes can be achieved by relying on social and legal conventions. Fost concludes that it is simply unnecessary to know whether brain dead patients are truly dead.[17]

There are, however, good reasons for defining death. Vital multiorgan transplantation requires death declaration to respect the dead-donor rule—the ethical axiom of vital multiorgan transplantation that bans killing an organ donor to procure organs even with the donor's consent.[18] Organized religions retain a great interest in the definition of death as evidenced by the ongoing rabbinic debate in Orthodox Judaism[19] and the recent Vatican study of the definition of death that culminated in the pronouncement of Pope John Paul II supporting the concept of brain death.[20] But the most compelling reason for defining death is to permit the drafting of successful public policies based on a scientifically accurate, coherent, and noncontrived biophilosophical formulation of human death. Laws governing physicians' declaration of death should be consistent with biological facts and not contrived for social purposes. It is true that societies may choose to make certain compromises on designating the legal time of death (such as whether to finesse the distinction between the "permanent" and "irreversible" loss of vital functions) that further a communal social good (allowing organ donation after cardiac death).[21] But agreement on a definition of death is essential for coherent and consistent public policy.

AREAS OF CONTROVERSY

Before defending a particular definition of death, it will be useful to review several persisting areas of controversy that obstruct the achievement of consensus on this issue. For the sake of simplicity, my discussion will be limited to the death of higher animals such as vertebrates, in whom death is a univocal phenomenon. That is, we mean the same thing by "death" when we say a man died as we do when we say a dog died. How one defines the death of a cell, organ, protozoan, or virus are valid biophilosophical questions, but they are not the topic of our attention here. This effort strives to make explicit the traditional meaning of "death" that is implicit in our ordinary consensual usage of the concept. This goal has become obscured by recent technology.

An analysis hoping to achieve consensus requires the consideration of nine controversial questions. When the analysis proceeds in the following logical order from the general to the specific, disagreements can be identified and clarified.

1. Is Death a Physical or Metaphysical Phenomenon?

Most writers claim that the answer to the question of whether an organism is dead can be settled by reference to physical facts alone. But this seemingly uncontroversial claim has been challenged. For example, Linda Emanuel appears to claim that death is a metaphysical phenomenon when she writes: "there is no state of death . . . to say 'she is dead' is meaningless because 'she' is not compatible with 'dead'."[22] And others have claimed that even if we knew all the relevant physical facts about a person or organism we still might not know whether it had died.[23]

2. Is Death a Biological Fact or an Arbitrary Social and Cultural Agreement?

Robert Veatch and Steven Miles argue that death determination is a social and cultural custom that can be contrived and modified based on personal preference, cultural practices, and religious beliefs.[24] Others disagree. They argue that because life is a biological phenomenon so must be its termination. On this view, while it is certainly true that social practices surrounding dying, death declaration, burial, and grieving are determined by culture, religion, law, and social norms, the event of death itself fundamentally is a fixed and immutable biological fact.

3. Does Death Pertain Directly to Human Organisms or to Persons?

Robert Lizza and Jeff McMahan hold that there are two types of death: death of the person and death of the organism. They argue that of these two, death of the person is the most important because we are our persons.[25] Against this view, it can be argued that what we mean by our consensual usage of the word "death" is the death of the human organism. Of course it is common to say "that person died," but by this usage we refer to the death of the human organism that was a person. Personhood is a psychosocial, spiritual, and legal concept based on a set of endowments, attributes, and qualities that are debatable. Personhood can be lost even when the human organism remains alive, but arguably, only organisms can die in a nonmetaphorical way.

4. Are There More Underlying States of an Organism Than Alive and Dead?

Amir Halevy and Baruch Brody claim that it is impossible to define death because there are transitional states of an organism between alive and dead that have features of both states.[26] Using the mathematical concept of fuzzy logic, they argue that alive and dead are fuzzy sets because dead and alive are mutually exclusive but not jointly exhaustive sets. They claim that whereas no organism can simultaneously and fully belong to both the set of living organisms and the set of dead organisms (mutually exclusive), some organisms can be in a condition in which they do not fully belong to either set (not jointly exhaustive). Against this formulation, it can be argued that because of limitations of current technology, we cannot confidently identify an organism's underlying state as clearly alive or dead, but this failure does not imply that the organism must be neither alive nor dead. Being alive and being dead could be mutually exclusive and jointly exhaustive sets. On this view, all organisms are either dead or alive; none is neither or both.

5. Is Death a Process or an Event?

In a famous exchange of opinions over thirty years ago, Robert Morrison argued that death was a process while Leon Kass argued that death was an event.[27] As Linda Emanuel showed, some deaths that follow a chronic, progressive illness with sequential organ failures comprise an apparent continuum in which it may seem arbitrary to delineate the precise moment of death.[28] But the transition from the state of alive to dead could be instantaneous, even though, for technical reasons, we may not be able to measure the change at the precise time it occurs. We may be able to determine the transition from alive to dead only in retrospect. Such a view is defended in a recent essay by Alan and Elisabeth Shewmon. They argue that death is an event and not a process using the rigorous mathematical analysis of state discontinuities that result from continuous changes in observable parameters. They conclude that the matter is closed and that further debates about death as an event or a process are "pointless."[29] But everyone agrees that dying and bodily disintegration are ineluctable processes. One way to settle the issue is to assert that death is the event that separates the process of dying from the process of bodily disintegration.

6. Is Death Reversible or Irreversible?

David Cole, arguing that death could be regarded as reversible, pointed out that "irreversible" can imply two separate meanings: irreversible by any foreseen future technology or irreversible using present technology.[30] If we conform to ordinary usage, we should choose Cole's second definition that the loss of critical function cannot be reversed using present technology. If future technology were to permit the loss of certain critical functions to become reversible, we would be forced to search for new irreversible critical functions upon which to rely. Restricting our attention to the secular account of mortals, it is impossible to return from the dead. The "near-death" experiences reported by some incipiently dying patients who were rescued from death at the last minute do not represent returning from the dead. Reported near-death experiences are simply memories recorded during an encephalopathy resulting from a disturbance of brain metabolism during incipient dying.[31]

7. At What Time Can Death Be Known to Occur?

Joanne Lynn and Ronald Cranford asserted that there are four possible choices for stating the time of death based on the loss of functions critical to life: "T1" when the critical function is lost; "T2" when the critical function is observed to be lost; "T3" when the critical function is irreversibly lost; and "T4" when the critical function is demonstrated to be irreversibly lost.[32] Assuming that death must be irreversible, the T1 and T2 times can be excluded. From a purely conceptual perspective, T3 represents the precise time of death. However, physicians must determine that death has occurred. Death may have occurred earlier, but physicians must perform testing to prove it before declaring a patient dead. Therefore, for practical reasons, it is most common for physicians to state the time of death as T4. The T4 time for death declaration is consistent with physicians' practices throughout the world and throughout history. Thus, by whatever tests are used, physicians determine the event of death primarily in retrospect.

There are two further areas of controversy, which I list below. Since they are essential to the definition of death that I will defend, they will be addressed in detail in the rest of the chapter.

8. *The Loss of Which Critical Functions is Most Relevant to a Definition of Death?*

9. *How Much Brain Function Must Be Lost for Death?*

A PARADIGM OF DEATH

In 1981, Charles Culver, Bernard Gert, and I proposed an approach to analyzing death that has been accepted by most subsequent scholars.[33] This approach proceeds from the conceptual and theoretical to the tangible and measurable.[34] It analyzes death in three sequential phases: (1) the philosophical task of determining the definition of death by making explicit the consensual concept of death; (2) the theoretical task of determining the criterion of death, i.e. a general standard or measurable condition that shows that the definition has been fulfilled; and (3) the medical task of determining tests of death for physicians to employ at the patient's bedside to demonstrate that the criterion of death has been fulfilled with no false positive and minimal false negative determinations.

This analytical approach to death is preceded by a series of preconditions, comprising what I call a "paradigm of death."[35] A paradigm of death is a set of conditions and assumptions that frame the discussion of the topic by identifying its nature, the class of phenomena to which it belongs, how it should be discussed, and its conceptual boundaries. The paradigm is designed to help identify areas of disagreement and lead to better understanding of grounds of controversy. Related to the areas of controversy reviewed in the previous section, the paradigm holds that death is a physical, univocal phenomenon. It is a biological fact that pertains directly to human organisms. It is an event that occurs when the functions critical to life are irreversibly lost. The paradigm holds that all human organisms are either dead or alive, and that death is irreversible.

THE DEFINITION OF DEATH

In light of this paradigm, I shall now turn to the definition of death. Several candidates for a formal definition of death have been proposed. An adequate definition should make explicit the consensual meaning of death that is implicit in our use of the concept.

In previous writings, Culver, Gert, and I have formally defined death as the cessation of functioning of the organism as a whole.[36] The organism as a whole represents that set of functions that is greater than the sum of its parts and that governs the interrelatedness and integration of its parts to provide the unity and wholeness of the organism. Organisms are not merely random collections of cells, tissues, and organs but have highly organized internal sequential functional hierarchies that are interrelated through emergent functions. An emergent function is a property of a whole not possessed by any of its component parts.[37] The functioning of the organism as a whole is operationalized through its emergent functions.

Death, on this definition, is the irreversible loss of those emergent functions responsible for the operation of the organism as a whole. The organism without its unifying emergent functions is merely a collection of independently functioning subsystems that individually or jointly may be able to be maintained mechanically by skilled physicians but whose unity, coherence, and wholeness have been forever lost.

Not everyone accepts this definition of death. Its main competitor—the higher brain formulation of death—was proposed by Robert Veatch over thirty years ago. Veatch argued that death should be defined formally as "the irreversible loss of that which is considered to be essentially significant to the nature of man."[38] He emphasized that it was the loss of man's consciousness and cognition served by the cerebral hemispheres that should count in a definition of human death, not the loss of integrating capacities served by lower brain structures. Veatch's definition was influential, and it attracted a loyal following of like-minded scholars who argued that the determination of brain death should be understood in terms of the higher-brain formulation of death.[39]

But the higher-brain formulation contains a fundamental flaw as a definition of death; namely, that it is not what we mean when we use the term "death." This is true for two reasons. First, it is not univocal because it is delineated solely for *homo sapiens*. Second, it implies that patients in an irreversible persistent vegetative state (PVS) are dead. Yet all societies, cultures, and laws consider PVS patients to be alive, despite their profound disability. It might be thought that declaring PVS patients dead is an attractive solution to the tragedy of these patients, since most people would not wish to continue to live if their consciousness and cognition were forever lost. But because there exist ethically and legally acceptable standards for withholding life-sustaining therapy from such patients to allow them to die, it is not necessary to assert that they are dead.

THE CRITERION OF DEATH

To be clinically useful, a definition of death must be supplemented by a criterion of death. A criterion of death is a general standard or measurable condition that shows that the definition of death has been fulfilled. There are two principal candidates for a criterion of death: irreversible absence of brain clinical functions and irreversible absence of circulation. I shall discuss each in turn.

The irreversible absence of brain clinical functions criterion—or brain-death criterion, for short—can refer to the functions of the whole brain, higher brain, or brain stem.[40] The whole-brain criterion requires the irreversible cessation of all clinical functions of the brain including the cerebral hemispheres, diencephalon (thalamus and hypothalamus), and brain stem. Advocates of a whole-brain criterion require widespread cessation of neuronal functions because each of these regions of the brain serves critical emergent functions responsible for the organism as a whole. The brain stem initiates and controls breathing, regulates circulation, and serves as the generator of conscious awareness through the ascending reticular activating system. The diencephalon provides the center for bodily homeostasis, regulating and coordinating neuroendocrine control systems such as those regulating body temperature, salt and water regulation, feeding behavior, and memory. Finally, the cerebral hemispheres serve an indispensable role in awareness that provides the conditions for all conscious behavior that serves the health and survival of the organism.

In assessing the whole-brain criterion of death it is important not to confuse clinical functions with cellular activities.[41] The whole-brain criterion requires the loss of brain clinical functions, not cellular activities. Thus, a continuation of functioning of some brain neurons that do not contribute to the brain's clinical functions remains compatible with the whole-brain criterion being satisfied. For example, EEG recordings of some brain-dead patients disclose measurable cellular activity.[42]

In part, confusion on this matter has resulted from the unnecessarily categorical language used in the Uniform Determination of Death Act (UDDA), a model death statute proposed by the President's Commission. The UDDA states, in part, "an individual who has sustained . . . irreversible cessation of all functions of the entire brain, including the brain stem, is dead."[43] Some scholars who have attacked the whole-brain criterion for not fulfilling the standards stipulated in the UDDA have erred by relying on the language of the UDDA without reading the explanation in the accompanying text. The explanation clarifies the distinction between functions and activities.[44]

The higher-brain criterion of death requires only the irreversible cessation of cerebral hemispheric function, which produces loss of consciousness and cognition. Clinical examples of conditions that would satisfy this criterion include the persistent vegetative state (PVS) and anencephaly.[45] In both conditions, patients have profound cerebral hemispheric destruction or absence producing loss of consciousness and cognition. But, according to the paradigm of death discussed above, the higher-brain formulation fails as a criterion of death because while it is undoubtedly necessary for death, it is not sufficient. Continued brain stem and hypothalamic functioning in PVS and anencephaly permit the continuation of many of the critical functions of the organism as whole. For years, a cadre of scholars and physicians has advocated converting to the higher-brain criterion.[46] But this change has not been endorsed by any jurisdiction or medical society because it is widely recognized that is incorrect to declare death on a person with spontaneous breathing and heartbeat who requires no mechanical organ support.

The brain stem criterion of death is satisfied by the irreversible loss of the capacities for breathing and consciousness. The brain stem alone is responsible for initiation and control of breathing through medullary respiratory centers, control of circulation through medullary vasomotor centers, and control of wakefulness through the pontine and midbrain portions of the ascending reticular activating system. Absence of brain stem functions produces utter coma and apnea. For these reasons, the United Kingdom has endorsed the brain stem criterion as the standard of death.[47]

In practice, the brain stem criterion is nearly congruent with the whole-brain criterion because both use the same bedside tests and in the vast majority of cases yield the same results.[48] The whole-brain and brain stem criteria use the same tests of death because the whole-brain criterion relies on absence of brain stem functioning to confirm that all brain clinical functions have ceased.[49] There are, however, both practical and theoretical shortcomings to the brain stem criterion. The practical shortcoming is that tests measuring brain electrical activity or absence of brain blood flow cannot be employed to confirm death as they can using a whole-brain criterion. The theoretical shortcoming is that by not requiring cessation of the clinical functions of the diencephalon or cerebral hemispheres, the brain stem criterion allows for the possibility of misdiagnosis of death. This could result from a pathological process that appears to destroy all brain stem activities, but that preserves a degree of conscious awareness that cannot be clinically detected. I have called such a possibility a "super locked-in syndrome."[50]

In a whimsical moment, Christopher Pallis, the leading advocate of the brain stem criterion, considered a similar possibility in a limerick that he remarked could have been penned by one of the *tricoteuses* (knitters) who sat by the guillotine in Paris in 1793, as memorably portrayed by Charles Dickens's character Madame LaFarge in *The Tale of Two Cities*.

> We knit on, too *blasées* to ask it:
>
> "Could the tetraparesis just mask it?
> When the brain stem is dead
> Can the cortex be said
> To tick on, in the head, in the basket?"[51]

Some scholars reject the brain-death criterion altogether. They favor the alternative mentioned above—the circulation criterion of death.

These scholars hold that death does not occur until the irreversible absence of systemic circulation. Brain-dead patients would be regarded as alive under a circulatory criterion. The circulation advocates defend their position on several grounds. First, even if they accept the definition of death as the cessation of functioning of the organism as a whole, they reject any brain criterion as showing that such a definition is satisfied.[52] Alan Shewmon, the most eloquent and prolific of the advocates of the circulation criterion, has shown that there are structures other than the brain (especially the spinal cord) that contribute to bodily subsystem integration. He claims that it is therefore erroneous to equate brain functions with such integration.[53] Shewmon also cites patients with what he has called "chronic" brain death, who were purportedly diagnosed as brain dead but whose ventilation and circulation were continued for months, or in one amazing case, for years.[54] He argues that it is counterintuitive to the concept of death for such prolonged visceral organ functioning to be possible and also for such patients to give birth to babies or grow. Therefore, he concludes, such patients must be alive.

I respond by acknowledging that, while not all body subsystem integration is carried out by the brain, the majority of the critical forms of integration that comprise emergent functions is performed by the brain. Accordingly, the irreversible loss of the brain's clinical functions is the death of the organism. The cases of "chronic" brain death represent technological *tours de force* indicative of the technical virtuosity of the modern intensive care unit. Absence of visceral organ functioning that is required by a circulatory criterion is unnecessary for death determination because it does not contribute to the functioning of the organism as a whole. The circulatory formulation fails as a criterion of death for the opposite reason as the higher brain formulation of the brain-death criterion. Whereas cessation of the higher brain functions is necessary but not sufficient for death, the cessation of circulatory functions is sufficient but not necessary for death.

For all these reasons, I believe that the correct criterion for death is the whole-brain formulation of the brain-death criterion.

THE TESTS OF DEATH

The President's Commission's Panel of Medical Consultants proposed tests for death which are consistent with the whole-brain death criterion

I have defended. These tests have been widely accepted.[55] The tests permit physicians to use the prolonged absence of breathing and heartbeat on the majority of deaths in which mechanical ventilation is not in place and resuscitation is not planned. The specific tests for brain death are employed only in the rare cases of hospitalized patients who are receiving mechanical ventilation. It is beyond the scope of this chapter to describe the tests to determine brain death, but the performance and validation of these bedside and confirmatory tests have been described elsewhere in detail.[56]

PUBLIC POLICY ON DEATH

The criterion of death can be incorporated as a standard in a death statute. In the United States, most enacted death statutes contain two parallel criteria: cardiopulmonary and brain based, comprising what Alexander Capron has called a bifurcated legal standard.[57] Parallel criteria permit physicians to determine death by either prolonged absence of cardiopulmonary function or absence of brain function. The Uniform Determination of Death Act (UDDA) proposed by the President's Commission is the prototype of a statute with a bifurcated legal standard.[58] The UDDA, or an adaptation of it, currently is law in nearly every state.[59]

Culver, Gert, and I criticized the UDDA on conceptual grounds shortly after it was proposed because it was based on a bifurcated criterion of death rather than a single brain criterion with bifurcated tests for death.[60] We pointed out that the reason the prolonged absence of cardiopulmonary function serves as an adequate standard for death is that it inevitably leads to the loss of brain function. We believed that it was important on conceptual grounds to state unequivocally that there was a single brain-based standard of death that physicians could test in two ways, depending on the clinical circumstance. But I now believe that such an end is less important given the UDDA's successful goal of creating a uniform death statute accepted across jurisdictions.

A major remaining public policy question is how much diversity of belief can or should be accommodated in a statute of death. In the United States, New Jersey amended its death statute in 1991 to provide a religious exemption to respect the beliefs of some residents, particularly a group of Orthodox Jews, whose religion did not accept brain death. The exemption prohibits physicians in New Jersey from using brain-based standards of death in a patient for whom it violated "personal religious beliefs or moral convictions."[61] New York later created administrative regulations to provide a similar, though more restricted, exemption.[62]

Some scholars have advocated that groups of believers or individuals have a liberty right to stipulate their own standard of death that should govern physicians' practices on them.[63] While I am in favor of respecting the rights of patients to make their own decisions with respect to consenting to or refusing life-sustaining therapy, I am skeptical about whether our society can tolerate a similar diversity of personal opinion about the determination of death. I support the laws granting religious exemptions, but believe it is desirable from a public policy perspective to preserve uniformity based upon consensus on a biophilosophically coherent formulation of death. Despite some valid points voiced by critics of the formulation of death defended in this chapter, it has achieved that consensus.

NOTES

1. Task Force on Death and Dying of the Institute of Society, Ethics, and the Life Sciences, "Refinements in the Criteria for the Determination of Death: An Appraisal," *Journal of the American Medical Association* 221 (1972): 48–53.

2. President's Commission for the Study of Ethical Problems in Medicine and Biomedical and Behavioral Research, *Defining Death: Medical, Legal and Ethical Issues in the Determination of Death* (Washington, D.C.: U.S. Government Printing Office, 1981).

3. The history of death determination up to the present technological era is chronicled in Martin S. Pernick, "Back from the Grave: Recurring Controversies over Defining and Diagnosing Death in History," in *Death: Beyond Whole-Brain Criteria*, ed. Richard M. Zaner (Dordrecht, the Netherlands: Kluwer Academic, 1988), 17–74.

4. The specific tests of death used by eighteenth- and nineteenth-century physicians are described in David J. Powner, Bruce M. Ackerman, and Ake Grenvik, "Medical Diagnosis of Death in Adults: Historical Contributions to Current Controversies," *The Lancet* 348 (1996): 1219–23.

5. See the discussion on this point in James L. Bernat, Charles M. Culver, and

Bernard Gert, "On the Definition and Criterion of Death," *Annals of Internal Medicine* 94 (1981): 389–94.

6. P. Mollaret and M. Goulon, "Le Coma Dépassé (Mémoire Préliminaire)," *Revue Neurologique* 101 (1959): 3–15.

7. "A Definition of Irreversible Coma: Report of the Ad Hoc Committee of the Harvard Medical School to Examine the Definition of Brain Death," *Journal of the American Medical Association* 205 (1968): 337–40.

8. Eelco F. M. Wijdicks, "Brain Death Worldwide: Accepted Fact but No Global Consensus in Diagnostic Criteria," *Neurology* 58 (2002): 20–25.

9. H. Richard Beresford, "Brain Death," *Neurologic Clinics* 17 (1999): 295–306.

10. See my review of religious views on brain death in James L. Bernat, *Ethical Issues in Neurology,* 2nd ed. (Boston: Butterworth-Heinemann, 2002), 257–60.

11. For example, Alexander Capron, the Executive Director of the President's Commission that published *Defining Death* (note 2), made this point in Alexander M. Capron, "Brain Death—Well Settled Yet Still Unresolved," *New England Journal of Medicine* 344 (2001): 1244–46.

12. See D. Alan Shewmon, "The Brain and Somatic Integration: Insights into the Standard Biological Rationale for Equating 'Brain Death' with Death," *Journal of Medicine and Philosophy* 26 (2001): 457–78; and D. Alan Shewmon, "The 'Critical Organ' for the Organism as a Whole: Lessons from the Lowly Spinal Cord," *Advances in Experimental Medicine and Biology* 550 (2004): 23–42.

13. Robert M. Taylor, "Re-examining the Definition and Criterion of Death," *Seminars in Neurology* 17 (1997): 265–70.

14. Robert D. Truog, "Is it Time to Abandon Brain Death?" *Hastings Center Report* 27, no. 1 (1997): 29–37.

15. For further scholarly rejections of brain death, see the entire issue of the *Journal of Medicine and Philosophy*, vol. 26 (2001); several articles in *The Definition of Death: Contemporary Controversies*, eds. Stuart J. Youngner, Robert M. Arnold, and Renie Schapiro (Baltimore, Md.: Johns Hopkins University Press, 1999); and a few articles in "Brain Death and Disorders of Consciousness," in *Advances in Experimental Medicine and Biology*, eds. Calixto Machado and D. Alan Shewmon, vol. 550 (New York: Kluwer Academic/Plenum Publishers, 2004).

16. For example, see Norman Fost, "The Unimportance of Death," in *The Definition of Death: Contemporary Controversies,* eds. Stuart J. Youngner, Robert M. Arnold, and Renie Schapiro (Baltimore, Md.: Johns Hopkins University Press, 1999), 160–78; and Stuart J. Youngner and Robert M. Arnold, "Philosophical Debates about the Definition of Death: Who Cares?" *Journal of Medicine and Philosophy* 26 (2001): 527–37.

17. Fost, "The Unimportance of Death," 161–62.

18. See the defense of the dead-donor rule in John A. Robertson, "The Dead Donor Rule," *Hastings Center Report* 29, no. 6 (1999): 6–14.

19. See the explanation of the rabbinic debate in Fred Rosner, "The Definition

of Death in Jewish Law," in *The Definition of Death: Contemporary Controversies*, eds. S. J. Youngner, R. M. Arnold, and R. Schapiro (Baltimore, Md.: Johns Hopkins University Press, 1999), 210–21.

20. In an August, 2000 address to the 18th Congress of the International Transplantation Society meeting in Rome, Pope John Paul II asserted that brain death was fully consistent with Catholic doctrine. For a detailed historical discussion of statements on brain death from Vatican academies, an account of the process of Vatican decision making, and an explanation of the Pope's statement, see Edward J. Furton, "Brain Death, the Soul, and Organic Life," *The National Catholic Bioethics Quarterly* 2 (2002): 455–70.

21. Declaring death in organ procurement after cardiac death protocols requires first waiting for five minutes of asystole or other ineffective cardiac rhythm. See Institute of Medicine, *Non-Heart-Beating Organ Transplantation: Practice and Protocols* (Washington, D.C.: National Academy Press, 2000), 22–24. When artificial resuscitation will not be attempted on such patients and we know they will not auto-resuscitate, it can be concluded that their loss of circulatory and respiratory function is permanent. But it may take many more minutes to prove that the loss is irreversible. For a discussion of the distinction between "permanent" and "irreversible," see Jeff McMahan, *The Ethics of Killing: Problems at the Margins of Life* (New York: Oxford University Press, 2002), 423–55.

22. Linda L. Emanuel, "Reexamining Death: The Asymptotic Model and a Bounded Zone Definition" *Hastings Center Report* 25, no. 4 (1995): 27–35.

23. Jeff McMahan, "The Metaphysics of Brain Death," *Bioethics* 9 (1995): 91–126. See also D. Parfit, *Reasons and Persons* (Oxford: Oxford University Press, 1990), 274–75.

24. Robert M. Veatch, "The Conscience Clause: How Much Individual Choice in Defining Death Can Our Society Tolerate?" in *The Definition of Death: Contemporary Controversies,* eds. Stuart J. Youngner, Robert M. Arnold, and Renie Schapiro (Baltimore, Md.: Johns Hopkins University Press, 1999), 137–60; and Steven Miles, "Death in a Technological and Pluralistic Culture," in *The Definition of Death: Contemporary Controversies,* eds. Stuart J. Youngner, Robert M. Arnold, and Renie Schapiro (Baltimore, Md.: Johns Hopkins University Press, 1999), 311–18.

25. See John P. Lizza, "Defining Death for Persons and Human Organisms," *Theoretical Medicine and Bioethics* 20 (1999): 439–53; and McMahan, "The Metaphysics of Brain Death."

26. See Amir Halevy and Baruch Brody, "Brain Death: Reconciling Definitions, Criteria, and Tests," *Annals of Internal Medicine* 119 (1993): 519–25; and Baruch Brody, "How Much of the Brain Must be Dead," in *The Definition of Death: Contemporary Controversies,* eds. Stuart J. Youngner, Robert M. Arnold, and Renie Schapiro (Baltimore, Md.: Johns Hopkins University Press, 1999), 71–82.

27. Robert S. Morison, "Death: Process or Event?" *Science* 173 (1971): 694–98; and Leon Kass, "Death as an Event: A Commentary on Robert Morison," *Science* 173 (1971): 698–702.

28. Emanuel, "Reexamining Death."

29. D. Alan Shewmon and Elisabeth S. Shewmon, "The Semiotics of Death and its Medical Implications," *Advances in Experimental Medicine and Biology* 550 (2004): 89–114.

30. David J. Cole, "The Reversibility of Death," *Journal of Medical Ethics* 18 (1992): 26–30.

31. S. Parnia and P. Fenwick, "Near Death Experiences in Cardiac Arrest: Visions of a Dying Brain or Visions of a New Science of Consciousness," *Resuscitation* 52 (2002): 5–11.

32. Joanne Lynn and Ronald E. Cranford, "The Persisting Perplexities in the Determination of Death," in *The Definition of Death: Contemporary Controversies,* eds. Stuart J. Youngner, Robert M. Arnold, and Renie Schapiro (Baltimore, Md.: Johns Hopkins University Press, 1999), 101–14.

33. This analysis is discussed in detail in Bernat, Culver, and Gert, "On the Definition and Criterion of Death." Alan and Elisabeth Shewmon recently claimed that our approach, though logical, is futile because language constrains our capacity to conceptualize life and death. They argue that death is an "ur-phenomenon [that is] conceptually fundamental in its class; no more basic concepts exist to which it can be reduced. It can only be intuited from our experience of it." See Shewmon and Shewmon, "The Semiotics of Death and its Medical Implications."

34. Our analysis followed the reasoning of an earlier proposal by Alexander Capron and Leon Kass that pointed out that agreement on a criterion of death first requires agreement on the concept of death. See Alexander M. Capron and Leon R. Kass, "A Statutory Definition of the Standards for Determining Human Death: An Appraisal and a Proposal," *University of Pennsylvania Law Review* 121 (1972): 87–118.

35. See my defense of the paradigm of death in James L. Bernat, "The Biophilosophical Basis of Whole-Brain Death," *Social Philosophy & Policy* 19, no 2. (2002): 324–42.

36. Bernat, Culver, and Gert, "On the Definition and Criterion of Death." In formulating this definition, we relied on the concept of organism as a whole that was introduced in 1916 by the biologist Jacques Loeb and that I subsequently rendered into more rigorous biophilosophical terms explaining how it provides the physiological basis for the coherent unity of the organism. See Jacques Loeb, *The Organism as a Whole* (New York: G. P. Putnam's Sons, 1916) and Bernat, "The Biophilosophical Basis of Whole–Brain Death."

37. Emergent functions are explained in M. Mahner and M. Bunge, *Foundations of Biophilosophy* (Berlin: Springer-Verlag, 1997), 29–30.

38. Robert M. Veatch, "The Whole Brain-Oriented Concept of Death: An Outmoded Philosophical Formulation," *Journal of Thanatology* 3 (1975): 13–30. He further refined his theory in subsequent articles including Robert M. Veatch, "Brain Death and Slippery Slopes," *Journal of Clinical Ethics* 3 (1992): 181–87; and Robert M. Veatch, "The Impending Collapse of the Whole-Brain Definition of Death," *Hastings Center Report* 23, no. 4 (1993): 18–24.

39. In addition to Robert Veatch, a number of scholars hold the higher-brain formulation of death. For example, see Michael B. Green and Daniel Wikler, "Brain Death and Personal Identity," *Philosophy and Public Affairs* 9 (1980): 105–33; Stuart J. Youngner and Edward T. Bartlett, "Human Death and High Technology: The Failure of the Whole Brain Formulation," *Annals of Internal Medicine* 99 (1983): 252–58; Karen G. Gervais, *Redefining Death* (New Haven, Conn.: Yale University Press, 1986); and Richard M. Zaner, ed., *Death: Beyond Whole-Brain Criteria* (Dordrecht, the Netherlands: Kluwer Academic, 1988).

40. I have compared and contrasted these positions in James L. Bernat, "How Much of the Brain Must Die in Brain Death?" *Journal of Clinical Ethics* 3 (1992): 21–26.

41. See Halevy and Brody, "Brain Death: Reconciling Definitions, Criteria, and Tests"; and Veatch, "The Impending Collapse of the Whole-Brain Definition of Death."

42. Residual EEG activity seen on unequivocally brain-dead patients has been described by Madeline M. Grigg, Michael A. Kelly, Gastone G. Celesia, Mona W. Ghobrial, and Emanuel R. Ross, "Electroencephalographic Activity after Brain Death," *Archives of Neurology* 44 (1987): 948–54.

43. See the discussion on this point by the President's Commission, cited in note 2, above, 72–73.

44. See President's Commission, *Defining Death*, 28–29, cited in note 2.

45. For authoritative descriptions of the persistent vegetative state and anencephaly, see Multi-Society Task Force on PVS, "Medical Aspects of the Persistent Vegetative State. Parts I and II," *New England Journal of Medicine* 330 (1994): 1499–1508, 1572–79; and Medical Task Force on Anencephaly, "The Infant with Anencephaly," *New England Journal of Medicine* 322 (1990): 669–74.

46. See works of scholars cited in notes 38 and 39.

47. See Conference of Medical Royal Colleges and their Faculties in the United Kingdom, "Diagnosis of Brain Death," *British Medical Journal* 2 (1976): 1187–88. See also the thorough explanation of the brain stem criterion in Christopher Pallis, *ABC of Brainstem Death*, 2nd ed. (London: British Medical Journal Publishers, 1995).

48. There are rare exceptions to this rule that are caused by primary brain stem disorders that selectively damage brain stem structures while sparing hemispheric structures. I have discussed these in Bernat, *Ethical Issues in Neurology*, 251–52.

49. I have explained the pathophysiological basis for this claim using the concepts of raised intracranial pressure and cerebral herniation in James L. Bernat, "A Defense of the Whole-Brain Concept of Death," *Hastings Center Report* 28, no. 2 (1998): 14–23.

50. The locked-in syndrome is a state of profound paralysis with preserved consciousness. Inexperienced examiners may wrongly conclude that the patient is unconscious. See Bernat, "How Much of the Brain Must Die in Brain Death?"

51. Christopher Pallis, *ABC of Brainstem Death* (London: British Medical Journal Publishers, 1983), 32.

52. Josef Seifert, "Is Brain Death Actually Death? A Critique of Redefinition of Man's Death in Terms of 'Brain Death,'" *The Monist* 76 (1993): 175–202.

53. Shewmon, "The Brain and Somatic Integration"; and Shewmon, "The 'Critical Organ' for the Organism as a Whole."

54. D. Alan Shewmon, "Chronic 'Brain Death': Meta-analysis and Conceptual Consequences," *Neurology* 51 (1998): 1538–45.

55. President's Commission, *Defining Death*, 159–166.

56. See, for example, Eelco F. M. Wijdicks, "The Diagnosis of Brain Death," *New England Journal of Medicine* 344 (2001): 1215–21.

57. Alexander M. Capron, "The Bifurcated Legal Standard for Determining Death: Does it Work?" in *The Definition of Death: Contemporary Controversies,* eds. Stuart J. Youngner, Robert M. Arnold, and Renie Schapiro (Baltimore, Md.: Johns Hopkins University Press, 1999), 117–36.

58. President's Commission, *Defining Death*, 72–81.

59. See the account of state statutes of death in the United States in Beresford, "Brain Death."

60. James L. Bernat, Charles M. Culver, and Bernard Gert, "Defining Death in Theory and Practice," *Hastings Center Report* 12, no. 1 (1982): 5–9.

61. See Robert S. Olick, "Brain Death, Religious Freedom, and Public Policy: New Jersey's Landmark Legislative Initiative," *Kennedy Institute of Ethics Journal* 4 (1991): 275–88.

62. See Beresford, "Brain Death."

63. See Robert A. Veatch, "The Conscience Clause: How Much Individual Choice in Defining Death Can Our Society Tolerate?" in *The Definition of Death: Contemporary Controversies,* eds. Stuart J. Youngner, Robert M. Arnold, and Renie Schapiro (Baltimore, Md.: Johns Hopkins University Press, 1999), 137–60; Dan W. Brock, "The Role of the Public in Public Policy on the Definition of Death," in *The Definition of Death: Contemporary Controversies*, eds. Stuart J. Youngner, Robert M. Arnold, and Renie Schapiro (Baltimore, Md.: Johns Hopkins University Press, 1999), 293–307; and Steven Miles, "Death in a Technological and Pluralistic Culture," *The Definition of Death: Contemporary Controversies*, eds. Stuart J. Youngner, Robert M. Arnold, and Renie Schapiro (Baltimore, Md.: Johns Hopkins University Press, 1999), 311–18.

II

FACING DEATH IN THE CLINIC

3

Against the Right to Die

J. David Velleman

In this chapter I offer an argument against establishing an institutional right to die, but I do not consider how my argument fares against countervailing considerations, and so I do not draw any final conclusion on the subject. The argument laid out in this chapter has certainly inhibited me from favoring a right to die, and it has also led me to recoil from many of the arguments offered for such a right. But I am very far from an all-things-considered judgment.

My argument is addressed to a question of public policy—namely, whether the law or the canons of medical practice should include a rule requiring, under specified circumstances, that caregivers honor a patient's request to be allowed or perhaps even helped to die. This question is distinct from the question whether anyone is ever morally entitled to be allowed or helped to die. I believe that the answer to the latter question is yes, but I doubt whether our moral obligation to facilitate some people's deaths is best discharged through the establishment of an institutional right to die.

I

Although I believe in our obligation to facilitate some deaths, I want to dissociate myself from some of the arguments that are frequently

49

offered for such an obligation. These arguments, like many arguments in medical ethics, rely on terms borrowed from Kantian moral theory—terms such as 'dignity' and 'autonomy.' Various kinds of life-preserving treatment are said to violate a patient's dignity or to detain him in an undignified state; and the patient's right of autonomy is said to require that we respect his competent and considered wishes, including a wish to die. There may or may not be some truth in each of these claims. Yet when we evaluate such claims, we must take care not to assume that terms like 'dignity' and 'autonomy' always express the same concepts, or carry the same normative force, as they do in a particular moral theory.

When Kant speaks, for example, of the dignity that belongs to persons by virtue of their rational nature, and that places them beyond all price,[1] he is not invoking anything that requires the ability to walk unaided, to feed oneself, or to control one's bowels. Hence the dignity invoked in discussions of medical ethics—a status supposedly threatened by physical deterioration and dependency—cannot be the status whose claim on our moral concern is so fundamental to Kantian thought. We must therefore ask whether this other sort of dignity, whatever it may be, embodies a value that's equally worthy of protection.

My worry, in particular, is that the word 'dignity' is sometimes used to dignify, so to speak, our culture's obsession with independence, physical strength, and youth. To my mind, the dignity defined by these values—a dignity that is ultimately incompatible with *being cared for* at all—is a dignity not worth having.[2]

I have similar worries about the values expressed by the phrase 'patient autonomy'; for there are two very different senses in which a person's autonomy can become a value for us. On the one hand, we can obey the categorical imperative, by declining to act for reasons that we could not rationally propose as valid for all rational beings, including those who are affected by our action, such as the patient. What we value in that case is the patent's capacity for self-determination, and we value it in a particular way—namely, by according it respect. We respect the patient's autonomy by regarding the necessity of sharing our reasons with him, among others, as a constraint on what decisions we permit ourselves to reach.

On the other hand, we can value the patient's autonomy by making it our goal to maximize his effective options. What we value, in that case, is not the patient's capacity but his opportunities for self-determination—his having choices to make and the means with which to implement them; and we value these opportunities for self-determination by regarding them as goods—as objects of desire and pursuit rather than respect.

These two ways of valuing autonomy are fundamentally different. Respecting people's autonomy, in the Kantian sense, is not just a matter of giving them effective options. To make our own decisions only for reasons that we could rationally share with others is not necessarily to give them decisions to make, nor is it to give them the means to implement their actual decisions.[3]

As with the term "dignity," then, we must not assume that the term "autonomy" is always being used in the sense made familiar by Kantian moral theory; and we must therefore ask ourselves what sort of autonomy is being invoked, and whether it is indeed something worthy of our moral concern. I believe that, as with the term "dignity," the answer to the latter question may be "no" in some cases, including the case of the right to die.

Despite my qualms about the use of Kantian language to justify euthanasia, I do believe that euthanasia can be justified, and on Kantian grounds. In particular, I believe that respect for a person's dignity, properly conceived, can require us to facilitate his death when that dignity is being irremediably compromised. I also believe, however, that a person's dignity can be so compromised only by circumstances that are likely to compromise his capacity for fully rational and autonomous decision making. So although I do not favor euthanizing people against their wills, of course, neither do I favor a policy of euthanizing people for the sake of deferring to their wills, since I think that people's wills are usually impaired in the circumstances required to make euthanasia permissible. The sense in which I oppose a right to die, then, is that I oppose treating euthanasia as a protected option for the patient.

One reason for my opposition is the associated belief (also Kantian) that so long as patients would be fully competent to exercise an option of being euthanized, their doing so would be immoral, in the majority of cases, because their dignity as persons would still be intact. I discuss this argument elsewhere, but I do not return to it in the present chapter.[4] In this chapter I discuss a second reason for opposing euthanasia as a protected option for the patient. This reason, unlike the first, is consequentialist.

What consequentialist arguments could there be against giving the option of euthanasia to patients? One argument, of course, would be that giving this option to patients, even under carefully defined conditions, would entail providing euthanasia to some patients for whom it would be a harm rather than a benefit.[5] But the argument that interests me does not depend on this strategy. My consequentialist worry about the right to die is not that some patients might mistakenly choose to die when they would be better off living.

In order to demonstrate that I am not primarily worried about mistaken requests to die, I shall assume, from this point forward, that patients are infallible, and that euthanasia would therefore be chosen only by those for whom it would be a benefit. Even so, I believe, the establishment of a right to die would harm many patients, by increasing their autonomy in a sense that is not only un-Kantian but also very undesirable.

This belief is sometimes expressed in public debate, although it is rarely developed in any detail. Here, for example, is Yale Kamisar's argument against "Euthanasia Legislation":

> Is this the kind of choice . . . that we want to offer a gravely ill person? Will we not sweep up, in the process, some who are not really tired of life, but think others are tired of them; some who do not really want to die, but who feel they should not live on, because to do so when there looms the legal alternative of euthanasia is to do a selfish or a cowardly act? Will not some feel an obligation to have themselves "eliminated" . . . ?[6]

Note that these considerations do not, strictly speaking, militate against euthanasia itself. Rather, they militate against a particular decision procedure for euthanasia—namely, the procedure of placing the choice of euthanasia in the patient's hands. What Kamisar is questioning in this particular passage is, not the practice of helping some patients to die, but rather the practice of asking them to choose whether to die. The feature of legalized euthanasia that troubles him is precisely its being an option offered to patients—the very feature for which it's touted, by its proponents, as an enhancement of the patient's autonomy. Kamisar's remarks thus betray the suspicion that this particular enhancement of one's autonomy is not to be welcomed.

But what exactly is the point of Kamisar's rhetorical questions? The whole purpose of giving people choices, surely, is to allow those choices to be determined by their reasons and preferences rather than ours. Kamisar may think that finding one's life tiresome is a good reason for dying whereas thinking that others find one tiresome is not. But if others honestly think otherwise, why should we stand in their way? Whose life is it anyway?

II

A theoretical framework for addressing this question can be found in Thomas Schelling's book *The Strategy of Conflict*[7] and in Gerald Dworkin's essay "Is More Choice Better Than Less?"[8] These authors have shown that our intuitions about the value of options are often mistaken, and their work can help us to understand the point of arguments like Kamisar's.

We are inclined to think that, unless we are likely to make mistakes about whether to exercise an option (as I am assuming we are not), the value of having the option is as high as the value of exercising it and no lower than zero. Exercising an option can of course be worse than nothing, if it causes harm. But if we are not prone to mistakes, then we will not exercise a harmful option; and we tend to think that simply having the unexercised option cannot be harmful. And insofar as exercising an option would make us better off than we are, having the option must have made us better off than we were before we had it—or so we tend to think.

What Schelling showed, however, is that having an option can be harmful even if we do not exercise it and—more surprisingly—even if we exercise it and gain by doing so. Schelling's examples of this phenomenon were drawn primarily from the world of negotiation, where the only way to induce one's opponent to settle for less may be by proving that one doesn't have the option of giving him more. Schelling pointed out that in such circumstances, a lack of options can be an advantage. The union leader who cannot persuade his membership to approve a pay cut, or the ambassador who cannot contact his head of state for a change of brief, negotiates from a position of strength; whereas the negotiator for whom all concessions are possible deals from weakness. If the rank and file give their leader the option of offering a pay cut, then management may not settle for anything less, whereas they might have settled for less if he hadn't had the option of making the offer. The union leader will then have to decide whether to take the option and reach an agreement or to leave the option and call a strike. But no matter which of these outcomes would make him better off, choosing it will still leave him worse off than he would have been if he had never had the option at all.

Dworkin has expanded on Schelling's point by exploring other respects in which options can be undesirable. Just as options can subject one to pressure from an opponent in negotiation, for example, they can subject one to pressure from other sources as well. The night cashier in a convenience store doesn't want the option of opening the safe—and not because he fears that he'd make mistakes about when to open it. It is precisely because the cashier would know when he'd better open the safe that his having the option would make him an attractive target for robbers; and it's because having the option would make him a target for robbers that he'd be better off without it. The cashier who finds himself opening the safe at gunpoint can consistently think that he's doing what's best while wishing that he'd never been given the option of doing it.

Options can be undesirable, then, because they subject one to various kinds of pressure; but they can be undesirable for other reasons, too. Offering someone an alternative to the status quo makes two outcomes possible for him, but neither of them is the outcome that was possible before. He can now choose the status quo or choose the alternative, but he can no longer *have* the status quo without *choosing* it. And having the status quo by default may have been what was best for him, even though choosing the status quo is now worst. If I invite you to a dinner party, I leave you the possibilities of choosing to come or choosing to stay away; but I deprive you of something that you otherwise would have had—namely, the possibility of being absent from my table by default, as you are on all other occasions. Surely, preferring to accept an invitation is consistent with wishing you had never received it. These attitudes are consistent because refusing to attend a party is a different outcome from *not* attending without having to refuse; and even if the former of these outcomes is worse than attending, the latter may still have been better. Having choices can thus deprive one of desirable outcomes whose desirability depends on their being unchosen.

The offer of an option can also be undesirable because of what it expresses. To offer a student the option of receiving remedial instruction after class is to imply that he is not keeping up. If the student needs help but doesn't know it, the offer may clue him in. But even if the student does not need any help, to begin with, the offer may so undermine his confidence that he will need help before long. In the latter case, the student may ultimately benefit from accepting the offer, even though he would have been better off not receiving it at all.

Note that in each of these cases, a person can be harmed by having a choice even if he chooses what's best for him. Once the option of offering a concession has undermined one's bargaining position, once the option of opening the safe has made one the target of a robbery, once the invitation to a party has eliminated the possibility of absence by default, once the offer of remedial instruction has implied that one needs it—in short, once one has been offered a problematic choice—one's situation has already been altered for the worse, and choosing what's best cannot remedy the harm that one has already suffered. Choosing what's best in these cases is simply a way of cutting one's losses.

Note, finally, that we cannot always avoid burdening people with options by offering them a second-order option as to which options they are to be offered. If issuing you an invitation to dinner would put you in an awkward position, then asking you whether you want to be invited would usually do so as well; if offering you the option of remedial instruction would send you a message, then so would asking you whether you'd like that option. In order to avoid doing harm, then, we are sometimes required, not only to withhold options, but also to take the initiative for withholding them.

III

Of course, the options that I have discussed can also be unproblematic for many people in many circumstances. Sometimes one has good reason to welcome a dinner invitation or an offer of remedial instruction. Similarly, some patients will welcome the option of euthanasia, and rightly so. The problem is how to offer the option only to those patients who will have reason to welcome it. Arguments like Kamisar's are best understood, I think, as warning that the option of euthanasia may unavoidably be offered to some who will be harmed simply by having the option, even if they go on to choose what is best.

I think that the option of euthanasia may harm some patients in all of the ways canvassed above; but I will focus my attention on only a few of those ways. The most important way in which the option of euthanasia may harm patients, I think, is that it will deny them the possibility of staying alive by default.

Now, the idea of surviving by default will be anathema to existentialists, who will insist that the choice between life and death is a choice that we have to make every day, perhaps every moment.[9] Yet even if there is a deep, philosophical sense in which we do continually choose to go on living, it is not reflected in our ordinary self-understanding. That is, we do not ordinarily think of ourselves or others as continually rejecting the option of suicide and staying alive by choice. Thus, even if the option of euthanasia won't alter a patient's existential situation, it will certainly alter the way in which his situation is generally perceived. And changes in the perception of a patient's situation will be sufficient to produce many of the problems that Schelling and Dworkin have described, since those problems are often created not just by having options but by *being seen* to have them.

Once a person is given the choice between life and death, he will rightly be perceived as the agent of his own survival. Whereas his existence is ordinarily viewed as a given for him—as a fixed condition with which he must cope—formally offering him the option of euthanasia will cause his existence thereafter to be viewed as his doing.

The problem with this perception is that if others regard you as choosing a state of affairs, they will hold you responsible for it; and if they hold you responsible for a state of affairs, they can ask you to justify it. Hence if people ever come to regard you as existing by choice, they may expect you to justify your continued existence. If your daily arrival in the office is interpreted as meaning that you have once again declined to kill yourself, you may feel obliged to arrive with an answer to the question, "Why not?"

I think that our perception of one another's existence as a given is so deeply ingrained that we can hardly imagine what life would be like without it. When someone shows impatience or displeasure with us, we jokingly say "Well, excuse me for living!" But imagine that it were no joke; imagine that the living were something for which one might reasonably be thought to need an excuse. The burden of justifying one's existence might make existence unbearable—and hence unjustifiable.

IV

I assume that people care, and are right to care, about whether they can justify their choices to others. Of course, this concern can easily seem like slavishness or neurotic insecurity; but it should not be dismissed too lightly. Our ability to justify our choices to the people around us is what enables us to sustain the role of rational agent in our dealings with them; and it is therefore essential to our remaining, in their eyes, an eligible partner in cooperation and conversation, or an appropriate object of respect.

Retaining one's status as a person among others is especially important to those who are ill or infirm. I imagine that when illness or infirmity denies one the rewards of independent activity, then the rewards of personal intercourse may be all that make life worth living. To the ill or infirm, then, the ability to sustain the role of rational person may rightly seem essential to retaining what remains of value in life. Being unable to account for one's choices may seem to entail the risk of being perceived as unreasonable—as not worth reasoning with—and consequently being cut off from meaningful intercourse with others, which is life's only remaining consolation.

Forcing a patient to take responsibility for his continued existence may therefore be tantamount to confronting with the following prospect: unless he can explain, to the satisfaction of others, why he chooses to exist, his only remaining reasons for existence may vanish.

V

Unfortunately, our culture is extremely hostile to any attempt at justifying an existence of passivity and dependence. The burden of proof will lie heavily on the patient who thinks that his terminal illness or chronic disability is not a sufficient reason for dying.

What is worse, the people with whom a patient wants to maintain intercourse, and to whom he therefore wants to justify his choices, are often in a position to incur several financial and emotional costs from any prolongation of his life. Many of the reasons in favor of his death are therefore likely to be exquisitely salient in their minds. I believe that some of these people may actively pressure the patient to exercise the option of dying. (Students who hear me say this usually object that no one would ever do such a thing. My reply is that no one would ever do such a thing as abuse his own children or parents—except that many people do.)

In practice, however, friends and relatives of a patient will not have to utter a word of encouragement, much less exert any overt pressure, once the option of euthanasia is offered. For in the discussion of a subject so hedged by taboos and inhibitions, the patient will have to make some assumptions about what they think and how they feel, irrespective of what they say.[10] And the rational assumption for him to make will be that they are especially sensible of the considerations in favor of his exercising the option.

Thus, even if a patient antecedently believes that his life is worth living, he may have good reason to assume that many of the people around him do not, and that his efforts to convince them will be frustrated by prevailing opinions about lives like his, or by the biases inherent in their perspective. Indeed, he can reasonably assume that the offer of euthanasia is itself an expression of attitudes that are likely to frustrate his efforts to justify declining it. He can therefore assume that his refusal to take the option of euthanasia will threaten his standing as a rational person in the eyes of friends and family, thereby threatening the very things that make his life worthwhile. This patient may rationally judge that he's better off taking the option of euthanasia, even though he would have been best off not having the option at all.

Establishing a right to die in our culture may thus be like establishing a right to duel in a culture obsessed with personal honor.[11] If someone defended the right to duel by arguing that a duel is a private transaction between consenting adults, he would have missed the point of laws against dueling. What makes it rational for someone to throw down or pick up a gauntlet may be the social costs of choosing not to, costs that result from failing to duel only if one fails to duel by choice. Such costs disappear if the choice of dueling can be removed. By eliminating the option of dueling (if we can), we eliminate the reasons that make it rational for people to duel in most cases. To restore the option of dueling would be to give people reasons for dueling that they didn't previously have. Similarly, I believe, to offer the option of dying may be to give people new reasons for dying.

VI

Do not attempt to refute this argument against the right to die by labeling it paternalistic. The argument is not paternalistic—at least, not in any derogatory sense of the word. Paternalism, in the derogatory sense, is the policy of saving people from self-inflicted harms, by denying them options that they might exercise unwisely. Such a policy is distasteful because it expresses a lack of respect for others' ability to make their own decisions.

But my argument is not paternalistic in this sense. My reason for withholding the option of euthanasia is not that others cannot be trusted to exercise it wisely. On the contrary, I have assumed from the outset that patients will be infallible in their deliberations. What I have argued is not that people to whom we offer the option of euthanasia might harm themselves but rather that in offering them this option, we will do them harm. My argument is therefore based on a simple policy of nonmalfeasance rather than on the policy of paternalism. I am arguing that we must not harm others by giving them choices, not that we must withhold the choices from them lest they harm themselves.

Of course, harming some people by giving them choices may be unavoidable if we could not withhold those choices from them without unjustly withholding the same choices from others. If a significant number of patients were both competent and morally entitled to choose euthanasia, then we might be obligated to make that option available even if, in doing so, we would inevitably give it to some who would be harmed by having it. Consider here a closely related option.[12] People are morally entitled to refuse treatment, because they are morally entitled not to be drugged, punctured, or irradiated against their wills—in short, not to be assaulted. Protecting the right not to be assaulted entails

giving some patients what amounts to the option of ending their lives.
And for some subset of these patients, having the option of ending their
lives by refusing treatment may be just as harmful as having the option
of electing active euthanasia. Nevertheless, these harms must be toler-
ated as an inevitable by-product of protecting the right not to be
assaulted.

Similarly, if I believed that people had a moral right to end their lives,
I would not entertain consequentialist arguments against protecting that
right. But I don't believe in such a moral right, for reasons to which I
have briefly alluded but cannot fully expound in this chapter. My willingness to entertain the arguments expounded here thus depends on
reasons that are explained elsewhere.[13]

VI

I have been assuming, in deference to existentialists, that a right to die
would not alter the options available to a patient but would, at most,
alter the social perception of his options. What would follow, however,
if we assumed that death was not ordinarily a genuine option? In that
case, offering someone the choice of euthanasia would not only cause
his existence to be perceived as his responsibility; it would actually
cause his existence to become his responsibility for the first time. And
this new responsibility might entail new and potentially burdensome
obligations.

That options can be undesirable because they entail obligations is a
familiar principle in one area of everyday life—namely, the practice of
offering, accepting, and declining gifts and favors. When we decline a
gift or a favor that someone has spontaneously offered, we deny him an
option, the option of providing us with a particular benefit. And our
reason for declining is often that he could not have the option of providing the benefit without being obligated to exercise that option. Indeed,
we sometimes feel obligated, on our part, to decline a benefit precisely
in order to prevent someone from being obligated, on his part, to provide it.[14] We thus recognize that giving or leaving someone the option
of providing a benefit to us may be a way of harming him, by burdening
him with an obligation.

When we decline a gift or favor, our would-be benefactor sometimes protests in language similar to that used by proponents of the right to die. "I know what I'm doing," he says, "and no one is twisting my arm. It's my money [or whatever], and I want you to have it." If he's unaware of the lurking allusion, he might even put it like this: "Whose money is it, anyway?"

Well, it is his money (or whatever); and we do believe that he's entitled to dispose of his money as he likes. Yet his right of personal autonomy in disposing of his money doesn't always require that we let him dispose of it on us. We are entitled—and, as I have suggested, sometimes obligated—to restrict his freedom in spending his money for our benefit, insofar as that freedom may entail burdensome obligations.

The language in which favors are declined is equally interesting as that in which they are offered. What we often say when declining a favor is, "I can't let you do that for me: it would be too much to ask." The phrase "too much to ask" is interesting because it is used only when we haven't in fact asked for anything. Precisely because the favor in question would be too much to ask, we haven't asked for it, and now our prospective benefactor is offering it spontaneously. Why, then, do we give our reason for not having solicited the favor as a reason for declining when it's offered unsolicited?

The answer, I think, is that we recognize how little distance there is between permitting someone to do us a favor and asking him to do it. Because leaving someone the option of doing us a favor can place him under an obligation to do it, it has all the consequences of asking for the favor. To say "I'm leaving you the option of helping me, but I'm not asking you to help" is to draw a distinction without a difference, since options can be just as burdensome as requests.

VIII

Clearly, a patient's decision to die will sometimes be a gift or a favor bestowed on loved ones whose financial or emotional resources are being drained by his condition. And clearly, death is the sort of gift that one might well want to decline, by denying others the option of giving it. Yet protections for the option of euthanasia would in effect protect the option of giving this gift, and they would thereby prevent the prospective beneficiaries from declining it. Establishing a right to die would thus be tantamount to adopting the public policy that death is never too much to ask.

I don't pretend to understand fully the ethics of gifts and favors. It's one of those subjects that gets neglected in philosophical ethics, perhaps because it has more to do with the supererogatory than the obligatory. One question that puzzles me is whether we are permitted to restrict people's freedom to benefit us in ways that require no active participation on our part. Someone cannot successfully give us a gift, in most cases, unless we cooperate by taking it into our possession; and denying someone the option of giving us a gift usually consists of refusing to do our part in the transaction. But what about cases in whch someone can do us a good turn without any cooperation from us? To what extent are we entitled to decline the favor by means of restrictions on his behavior rather than omissions in ours?

Another question, of course, is whether we wouldn't, in fact, play some part in the deaths of patients who received socially sanctioned euthanasia. Would a medically assisted or supervised death be a gift that we truly took no part in accepting? What if "we"—the intended beneficiary of the gift—were society as a whole, the body that established the right to die and trained physicians in its implementation? Surely, establishing the right to die is tantamount to saying, to those who might contemplate dying for the social good, that such favors will never be refused.

These considerations, inconclusive though they are, show how the theoretical framework developed by Schelling and Dworking might support remarks like Kamisar's about patients' "obligation to have themselves 'eliminated.'" The worry that a right to die would become an obligation to die is of a piece with other worries about euthanasia, not in itself, but as a problematic option for the patient.

IX

As I have said, I favor euthanasia in some cases. And of course, I believe that euthanasia must not be administered to competent patients without their consent. To that extent, I think that the option of dying will have to be presented to some patients, so that they can receive the benefit of a good death.

On the basis of the foregoing arguments, however, I doubt whether policymakers can formulate a general definition that distinguishes the circumstances in which the option of dying would be beneficial from those in which it would be harmful. The factors that make an option problematic are too subtle and too various to be defined in a statute or regulation. How will the option of euthanasia be perceived by the patient and his loved ones? How will it affect the relations among them? Is he likely to fear being spurned for declining the option? Would he exercise the option merely as a favor to them? And are they genuinely willing to accept that favor? Sensitivity to these and related questions could never be incorporated into an institutional rule defining conditions under which the option must be offered.

Insofar as I am swayed by the foregoing arguments, then, I am inclined to think that society should at most permit, and never require, health professionals to offer the option of euthanasia or to grant patients' requests for it. We can probably define some conditions under which the option should never be offered; but we are not in a position to define conditions under which it should always be offered; and so we can at most define a legal permission rather than a legal requirement to offer it. The resulting rule would leave caregivers free to withhold the option whenever they see fit, even if it is explicitly and spontaneously requested. And so long as caregivers are permitted to withhold the option of euthanasia, patients will not have a right to die.

X

The foregoing arguments make me worry even about an explicitly for-mulated permission for the practice of euthanasia, since an explicit law or regulation to this effect would already invite patients, and hence potentially pressure them, to request that the permission be exercised in their case. I feel most comfortable with a policy of permitting euthana-sia by default—that is, by a tacit failure to enforce the institutional rules that currently serve as barriers to justified euthanasia, or a gradual elim-ination of those rules without fanfare. The best public policy of eutha-nasia, I sometimes think, is no policy at all.

This suggestion will surely strike some readers as scandalous, because of the trust that it would place in the individual judgment of physicians and patients. But I suspect that to place one's life in the hands of another person, in the way that one does today when placing oneself in the care of a physician, may simply be to enter a relationship in which such trust is essential, because it cannot be replaced or even underwritten by institutional guarantees. Although I do not share the conventional view that advances in medical technology have outrun our moral understanding of how they should be applied, I am indeed tempted to think they have outrun the capacity of institutional rules to regulate their application. I am therefore tempted to think that public policy regulating the relation between physician and patient should be weak and vague by design; and that insofar as the aim of medical ethics is to strengthen or sharpen such policy, medical ethics itself is a bad idea.

NOTES

This essay is reproduced with revision from J. David Velleman, "Against the Right to Die," *The Journal of Medicine and Philosophy* 17, no. 6 (1992): 665–81. Reprinted by permission of Taylor & Francis, Inc., www.taylorandfrancis.com.

The essay began as a comment of a paper by Dan W. Brock, presented at the Central Division of the APA in 1991. See Dan W. Brock, "Voluntary Active Euthanasia," *Hastings Center Report* 22 (March–April 1992): 10–22. I received help in writing that paper from Dan W. Brock, Elizabeth Anderson, David Hills, Yale Kamisar, and Patricia White. The present version of the essay replaces sections II and III of the original paper with a new and substantially different section II.

1. I. Kant, *Groundwork of the Metaphysic of Morals,* trans. H. J. Paton (New York: Harper and Row, 1964), 102.

2. Here I echo some excellent remarks on the subject by Felicia Ackerman, "No, Thanks, I Don't Want to Die with Dignity," *Providence Journal-Bulletin*, April 19, 1990. I discuss the issue of "dying with dignity" in J. David Velleman, "A Right of Self-Termination?" *Ethics* 109 (1999): 606–28.

3. I discuss this issue further in J. David Velleman, "Love as a Moral Emotion," *Ethics* 109 (1999): 338–74 (see 356–58, esp. notes 69, 72).

4. Velleman, "A Right of Self-Termination?"

5. Yale Kamisar, "Euthanasia Legislation: Some Non-religious Objections," in *Euthanasia and the Right to Death: The Case for Voluntary Euthanasia,* ed. A. B. Downing (New York: Humanities Press, 1970), 85–133.

6. Kamisar, "Euthanasia Legislation," 85–133.

7. Thomas Schelling, *The Strategy of Conflict* (Cambridge, Mass.: Harvard University Press, 1960).

8. Gerald Dworkin, "Is More Choice Better Than Less?" *Midwest Studies in Philosophy* 7 (1982): 47–61.

9. The locus classicus for this point is of course Albert Camus' essay "The Myth of Sisyphus," in *The Myth of Sisyphus and Other Essays,* trans. Justin O'Brien (New York: Vintage Books, 1959).

10. Thomas Schelling, "Strategic Relationships in Dying," in *Choice and Consequence* (Cambridge, Mass.: Harvard University Press, 1984).

11. For this analogy, see Lance K. Stell, "Dueling and the Right to Life," *Ethics* 90 (1979): 7–26. Stell argues—implausibly, in my view—that one has the right to die for the same reason that one has a right to duel.

12. The analogy is suggested in the form of an objection to my arguments, by Dan W. Brock, "Voluntary Active Euthanasia," *Hastings Center Report* 22 (March–April 1992): 10–22; and reprinted in *Life and Death: Philosophical Essays in Biomedical Ethics* (Cambridge: Cambridge University Press, 1993).

13. See Velleman, "A Right of Self-Termination?"

14. Of course, there are many other reasons for declining gifts and favors, such as pride, embarrassment, or a desire not to be in someone else's debt. My point is simply that there are cases in which these reasons are absent and a very different reason is present—namely, our desire not to burden someone else with obligations.

4

The Skull at the Banquet

David Barnard

—Doctor, Doctor, will I die?
—Yes, my dear. And so will I.

ANNE

Anne's breast cancer had metastasized aggressively, and she was dying. We have a description of her dying days from Michael Kearney, who helped care for her at a hospice in Dublin where Kearney was a consultant in palliative medicine. Kearney included his narrative of Anne's death in his book *Mortally Wounded: Stories of Soul Pain, Death, and Healing.*[1]

Anne was a young mother of three boys. She and her husband, John, had been separated for two years. One year after surgery for her breast cancer the disease was found to have spread to her lungs, her bones, and her liver. Her oncologist offered further chemotherapy, but Anne declined. Her goal now, she told Kearney when he visited her in her hospital room, was to maintain the best possible quality of life, because, as she said, "there is so much I want to do, for myself and for my children." It was apparent to Kearney from this conversation that Anne's pain at her separation from John was still raw and that it had taken a serious emotional toll on the boys as well. Kearney assured Anne that his palliative care team would help her with her physical symptoms and that the social worker could try to help with some of the family issues.

Three months later Anne was readmitted to the hospital with extreme breathlessness. Doctors inserted a chest tube to draw off the fluid that had accumulated around her lungs. When Kearney visited this time, Anne told him of terrifying nightmares and intense anxiety. Kearney offered to spend time with Anne during her hospitalization to explore her feelings and fears. He was adept at imagework and guided visualization techniques, and these sessions appeared to help Anne find a measure of peace. She was stunned a day or two later, however, when one of her doctors, in reply to Anne's question about the medical usefulness of the chest tubes, replied, "Have you ever thought about a move to the hospice?"

Despite Anne's resentment of this doctor's abruptness, she discussed the hospice idea with Kearney later that day and came to feel that she wanted to make the move. Two days later Anne moved to the hospice unit, which was staffed by a large and experienced multidisciplinary palliative care team. For most of her time there, the team succeeded in controlling the most distressing of Anne's physical symptoms. Her imagework and conversations with Kearney, meanwhile, appeared to enlarge her capacity to acknowledge and express her fears and regrets over her impending death. She also experienced some periods of relief from the anxiety that gnawed at her about the fate of her three boys, though she was not completely free of nightmares. Her parents and sisters spent a lot of time at the hospice, sitting at Anne's bedside or gathered in a dayroom nearby.

Two days before she died, Anne became restless, agitated, and increasingly short of breath. She declined Kearney's offer of more medication to alleviate the shortness of breath, saying it made her too sleepy. She went in and out of consciousness and often seemed confused. Kearney checked on her from time to time and tried to reassure Anne's family. He told them that Anne's physical symptoms were relatively well controlled and that he thought she had "prepared as much as anyone could, for whatever was ahead." Kearney's assessment was a reflection, among other things, of the accomplishments of the palliative care team and of his own skill and attentiveness as Anne's physician. The next day, however, by his own later admission, Kearney made a mistake.

Anne awoke that morning in great confusion and anxiety. As Kearney described the scene,

When I went into her room a nurse was sitting beside a distraught-looking Anne attempting to reassure her. Meanwhile Anne, wide-eyed and kneeling on her bed, was calling out and rummaging through the sheets "looking for my baby." I pulled a chair over so I was facing Anne, took her hand, and said, "Anne, it's okay. We are with you. It's okay. It's going to be all right." At that she stopped her searching for a moment, looked at me as if I were a stranger, and clearly and slowly, with the annoyance of one talking to another who despite repeated attempts could not be made to understand, said, "It's *not* all right." I sat silently for a while. Then I said, "Let go to your body, Anne. Let your body rest now. Let go to the tiredness." She lay back against her pillows and began to settle. Her family was nearby all day, coming in and out of her room. Late in the afternoon she once again became restless and agitated and did not settle with reassurance. I decided she needed an injection to help her relax. Shortly after having this, she went back to sleep. During her final hours Anne remained asleep with her three sons, her sisters, and her brothers at her bedside. She died early that evening.[2]

In his later reflection on Anne's story, Kearney commented that Anne's last words of rebuke were justified. He had, with his well-meaning reassurance, failed to acknowledge to her "the enormity of what she was living." He felt he had trivialized the anguish of "a young woman looking back at me over her shoulder as she stood alone on the threshold of death's dark kingdom."[3] We can appreciate the force of Kearney's self-criticism, but we can also sympathize with his predicament as he sat beside Anne's bed. He was, after all, a witness to Anne's crossing of the threshold. He had accompanied her toward death with attentiveness, patience, and skill. He had journeyed with her, through their intense imagework sessions, into the depths of her fears of abandonment and loss and helped her make connections to spiritually revivifying memories of her family's love for her and to the sense of Jesus's love. He had done all this, only to be confronted now with Anne's terror, and his own helplessness. Anne had seemed to respond gratefully in the past to those very words, "We are with you. It is okay." Why not now?

Kearney did something else while he was at Anne's bedside that day, but unlike his ill-timed repetition of reassuring words, it passes without comment from him. "I decided she needed an injection to help her relax. Shortly after having this, she went back to sleep. During her final hours Anne remained asleep. . . . She died early that evening."

On first reading, Kearney's act of sedating Anne seems to be profoundly compassionate. With the luxury of hindsight and a reader's complete detachment from the clinical moment, however, two questions arise. Why did Kearney think then that Anne needed to relax? Why did he believe he should decide this by himself? Both judgments seem uncharacteristic.

Throughout the narrative (and throughout his book) Kearney emphasizes the spiritual and psychological value to people of moving directly toward the center of their feelings of anguish or despair—what he calls "soul pain"—and the importance of accompanying them into that place of suffering. Only the day before, Anne herself had told Kearney not to medicate her to alleviate her breathlessness because she wanted to stay awake and alert, and Kearney had acceded to her request. Had he concluded that now Anne's restlessness was nothing other than "terminal agitation" devoid of psychological or spiritual content, and therefore there was no point in remaining with her as a companion in her existential suffering?

Throughout his narrative (and throughout his book) Kearney is meticulous in his devotion to wide consultation with his team and to shared decision making with his patients. At this moment, however, he acted unilaterally on his perception that Anne should be sedated into unconsciousness. Did the moment seem particularly urgent? Did Kearney wish to spare the family members (who were close by in the dayroom) the stress of sharing in his decision making at a moment such as this? Did he believe the judgment required was uniquely medical?[4]

Affirmative answers to all of these questions add up to a plausible scenario: Anne, clearly close to death, was tossing restlessly and seemingly beyond verbal comfort. Her tired family waited anxiously for the end to come. Her physician, recognizing the signs of "agitated delirium," was able to use his knowledge and his medicines to provide everyone precious final hours of bedside peace.

But another scenario also suggests itself. In this admittedly speculative scenario (but then, the first scenario is speculative also), Kearney's customary approach to patients and their suffering was thoroughly discombobulated by overwhelming forces swirling around him, forces set loose by Kearney's existential encounter with death. Sitting face-to-face with Anne on the threshold of death's dark kingdom was too much, even for an experienced and self-aware physician like Michael Kearney to bear, without his having to retreat into self-protective platitudes

("It's going to be all right") and projecting his intense anxiety onto his patient ("she needed an injection to help her relax").

PALLIATIVE CARE TRIUMPHALISM

The point of emphasizing this alternative scenario is not to criticize Kearney or to fault his treatment of Anne. Looked at as a whole, Anne's experience at the hospice exemplified palliative care at its best. Her experience of dying was almost certainly better in that setting than had she spent her last weeks or months in and out of acute hospital wards, negotiating her difficult family situation, her emotional turmoil, and the side effects of additional rounds of chemotherapy. Rather, the alternative scenario calls attention to an aspect of caring for the dying that deserves greater emphasis than it typically receives: the power of the direct encounter with death—in the guise of the death of the patient—to disrupt the carer's relationship and communication with the dying person, fluster ordinarily rational decision making, and capsize the palliative care team's carefully wrought treatment plans.

This aspect is all too often obscured by a certain triumphalist tendency of the contemporary field of palliative care. This is the tendency to equate palliative medicine's growing sophistication in symptom management and in the orchestration of the dying process according to various pharmacological, psychological, and social protocols, with mastery of the problem of death. Kearney himself has been an important critic of this tendency. He has warned in particular that palliative medicine is in danger of focusing too narrowly on its growing prowess in controlling physical symptoms, at the expense of a broader engagement—less certain of success—with spiritual and existential suffering.[5]

A hollowness at the base of palliative care triumphalism reveals itself when the physician, nurse, or other carer comes face to face with the uncontrollable power of death. That power can cause even the most carefully arranged system of care to buckle. Advance directives are unavailable or they are perceived to be too vague to be of use; or people's ambivalence at the prospect of dying delays a focus on palliative care until the pain and indignity that people say they want to avoid have already happened. That power can cause even the most accomplished and experienced carers to flinch. They are then apt to retreat into self-protective emotional distancing or to deploy aggressive but fruitless medical technology to assuage their helplessness.

Palliative care triumphalism also obscures an uncomfortable truth about the care of the dying in the United States: it has not improved very much in the last three decades. Many will take issue with this judgment. They will point to the spread of living wills and advance directives (though their efficacy in helping people avoid unwanted treatment at the end of life is highly debatable).[6] They will cite statistics on the greater numbers of people who now enroll in hospice (though hospice lengths of stay have dropped in the last ten years with the median now hovering around twenty-five days).[7] And they will emphasize the increase in the number of hospitals with palliative care programs (although no more than 14 percent of United States hospitals reported having one in the latest national survey).[8]

Even if we accept these claims in their most positive light, it is instructive and sobering to compare two assessments of the care of the dying written approximately thirty years apart.

The first, by Eric Cassell, was published in 1974:

> We have seen how the care of the terminally ill has changed in the United States. They are older now and die more frequently in institutions. But that bare frame of facts conceals increasing distress within the society over the quality of their dying. When death occurs in the modern hospital there seems to be more concern for the disease than for the dying person, more concern for life as a succession of heartbeats, than life as meaning. When death occurs in nursing homes it is as if life just dribbled out—custodial care seemingly inconvenienced by individual difference or tenacity for life.[9]

In the three decades since Cassell wrote those words we have witnessed the growth of the advance directive movement, the hospice movement, and the palliative care movement. In the past ten years alone the Robert Wood Johnson Foundation has committed more than $148 million, and the Open Society Institute's Project on Death in America has committed $45 million to improving end-of-life care in the United States—to cite only the most active funders in this area.[10] And yet, here is how an official report from the Institute of Medicine described the care of people with advanced cancer in 2001:

> For at least half of those dying of cancer—most of them elderly and many vulnerable—death entails a spectrum of symptoms, including pain, labored

breathing, distress, nausea, confusion, and other physical and psychological conditions that go untreated or undertreated and vastly diminish the quality of their remaining days. The patient is not the only one who suffers during the dying process. The impact on families and caregivers is still poorly documented, but evidence had begun to be collected demonstrating a heavy and mostly unrelieved emotional and financial burden. . . . A major problem in palliative care is the underrecognition, underdiagnosis, and thus undertreatment of patients with significant distress, ranging from existential anguish to anxiety and depression. This situation continues to exist despite the fact that when dying patients themselves have been asked their primary concerns about their care, three of their five concerns were psychosocial: (1) no prolongation of dying; (2) maintaining a sense of control; and (3) relieving burdens (conflicts) and strengthening ties.[11]

Perhaps we should not make too much of the similarity between these two assessments. After all, the care of the dying reflects wider aspects of culture and society, and cultural and social changes take time. As for those millions of dollars from the Robert Wood Johnson Foundation and Project on Death in America, much of that money has been directed at reforming medical education, developing a new generation of palliative care specialists, and encouraging community and statewide initiatives to improve end-of-life care. These are long-term investments whose impact will not be measurable for some time. Yet it is just this expectation—that we have only to wait for these investments in palliative care infrastructure and clinical skills to take hold in order to solve the problems of the dying—that Kearney's experience with Anne calls into question.

A caution is immediately in order to prevent misunderstanding. It is impossible to overstate the importance of palliative care in the management of the physical, psychological, and social distress of the dying and their families. A scandal of modern medical care is the gap between the state of the art in pain and symptom management and the quality of care that is actually received by millions of people every year who are never referred to skilled providers, or who are referred too late in their dying process to receive significant benefit. Efforts to expand and refine the evidence base for palliative care interventions are proceeding apace. These efforts are indispensable and overdue. Triumphalism begins to distort the picture, however, when our proliferating techniques for easing the process of dying are confused with the means to protect patients and carers from the de-centering, disruptive power of death.

THE SICK SOUL

Many people believe that making dying easier *does* protect us from the power of death, or at least the only aspect of its power that living people should care very much about. They agree with Woody Allen when he said, "I'm not afraid of death. I just don't want to be there when it happens." In other words, death itself is not the enemy, only all of the painful and frightening things that can happen while a person is actually dying. Once we know those will be successfully managed, we should be able to face the prospect of death itself—that is, being dead—with equanimity. As Kathleen Foley, Director of the Project on Death in America has put it, "Death is inevitable, but severe suffering is not."[12] This is the official philosophy of hospice: death is "a natural part of life," and "acceptance"—not denial, not anger, not fear—is the ideal attitude for the dying and those who care for them. This is also the philosophy that Philippe Ariès refers to—with considerable irony—at the very end of his monumental study, *The Hour of Our Death*. For Ariès, the modern effort to "accept" death actually rests on a historically conditioned form of denial. It depends on purging the concept of death of its ancient association with evil. The modern attitude was promoted, Ariès writes, by

a small elite of anthropologists, psychologists, and sociologists . . . [who] acknowledge the necessity of death, but . . . want it to be accepted and no longer shameful. Although they may consult the ancient wisdom, there is no question of turning back or of rediscovering the evil that has been abolished. They propose to reconcile death with happiness. Death must simply become the discreet but dignified exit of a peaceful person from a helpful society that is not torn, not even overly upset by the idea of a biological transition without significance, without pain or suffering, and ultimately without fear.[13]

A profound optimism underlies the expectation that our increasing success at managing the physical and psychological distress of dying will (or at least can) ultimately banish the fear of death. It calls to mind what William James identified as the religion of "healthy-mindedness." James saw the traces of this metaphysical optimism, which he called the American people's "only decidedly original contribution to the systematic philosophy of life,"[14] in a wide range of social and religious

phenomena of his day, from the mind-cure movement to liberal Protes-
tantism. In James's paraphrase of the proponents of the mind cure,

> What can be more base and unworthy than the pining, puling, mumping
> mood, no matter by what outward ills it may have been engendered? What is
> more injurious to others? What less helpful way out of the difficulty? It but
> fastens and perpetuates the trouble that occasioned it and increases the total
> evil of the situation. At all costs, then, we ought to reduce the sway of that
> mood; we ought to scout it in ourselves and others and never show it toler-
> ance.[15]

James thought that the wide popularity of the liberal Christian
churches in late nineteenth-century America:

> might fairly be called a victory of healthy-mindedness within the church over
> the morbidness with which the old hell-fire theology was more harmoniously
> related. We have now whole congregations whose preachers, far from magni-
> fying our consciousness of sin, seem devoted rather to making little of it.
> They ignore, or even deny, eternal punishment and insist on the dignity rather
> than on the depravity of man. They look at the continual preoccupation of the
> old-fashioned Christian with the salvation of his soul as something sickly and
> reprehensible, rather than admirable; and a sanguine and "muscular" attitude,
> which to our forefathers would have seemed purely heathen, has become in
> their eyes an ideal element of Christian character.[16]

James admired healthy-mindedness. Not only does it comport with
much in human nature, it also supplies vital motivation for projects that
bring about much individual and social good. So, too, has optimism
about the potential of skilled palliative care to ease the process of dying
stimulated progress in symptom management and encouraged imaginative schemes for the organization and financing of end-of-life care.

But James was careful to set the optimistic religion of "healthy-
mindedness" alongside another worldview, that of "the sick soul." To
the sick soul, evil is so radically enmeshed in the universal fabric that
human reason and creativity, no matter how robust, will not avail
against it. An extraordinary supernatural remedy is humanity's only
hope. Though James gave each worldview approximately equal time
and lavished his customary eloquence upon both, the sick soul's attitude seems particularly convincing. The sick soul believes that healthy-
mindedness rests on willful self-deception. To remain metaphysically

or theologically optimistic in the face of disease, death, and destruction actually requires that "we divert our attention from [them] as much as we can; and the slaughterhouses and indecencies without end on which our life is founded are huddled out of sight and never mentioned, so that the world we recognize officially in literature and in society is a poetic fiction far handsomer and cleaner and better than the world that really is."[17]

To the sick soul, this illusion must finally give way to a more sober but ultimately more productive question: "whether pity, pain, and fear, and the sentiment of human helplessness may not open a profounder view and put into our hands a more complicated key to the meaning of the situation."[18] Or, in James's typically vivid phrase,

Let sanguine healthy-mindedness do its best with its strange power of living in the moment and ignoring and forgetting, still the evil background is really there to be thought of, and the skull will grin in at the banquet.[19]

THE EXISTENTIAL MOMENT

In the setting of end-of-life care, the skull at the banquet is the felt awareness that we, too, will die. This has nothing to do with the abstract acknowledgment that "death is inevitable," as taught by the syllogism that Tolstoy's Ivan Ilych learned in grade school:

[To Ivan, recalling his schoolboy logic lesson as he lay dying,] "Caius is a man, men are mortal, therefore Caius is mortal," had always seemed to him correct as applied to Caius but certainly not as applied to himself. That Caius—man in the abstract—was mortal, was perfectly correct, but he was not Caius, not an abstract man but a creature quite, quite separate from all others. He had been little Vanya, with a mamma and a papa, with Mitya and Volodya, with the toys, a coachman, and a nurse, and afterwards with Katenka and with all the joys, griefs, and delights of childhood, boyhood, and youth. . . . "Caius really was mortal, and it was right for him to die; but for me, little Vanya, Ivan Ilych, with all my thoughts and emotions, it's altogether a different matter. It cannot be that I ought to die. That would be too terrible."[20]

Balfour Mount describes the jolt this awareness administers to our sense of reality as "the existential moment," wherein "we are sucked into the startling realization that the rules of the game are not what we had imagined. Not only does life depend on unfamiliar rules, it never *was* defined by the terms we had always held to be reliable."[21] Among the reactions this awareness is likely to provoke are the feelings of helplessness and anger that, according to the second scenario sketched above, attended Michael Kearney's last encounters with Anne.

Reactions such as these have often been noted by commentators on the doctor-patient relationship in the setting of terminal illness. The psychiatrist John Hinton, for example, who conducted groundbreaking work on the psychology of dying in association with Cicely Saunders and St. Christopher's Hospice in London, observed (perhaps with a touch of British understatement):

> To the dying person his doctor, however much he is trusted and regarded as a source of treatment, is no longer one with the power to cure; to the doctor, the patient has become one whose death, despite every possible effort, he is impotent to prevent. This gives rise to problems in the special professional relationship that often develops between a patient and his doctor and besides that, they have the difficulties that face any two people trying to adjust to the fact that one of them is shortly going to die.[22]

Steven Miles and Robert Burt have both emphasized that unacknowledged, irrational impulses stirred up by the patient's nearness to death are likely to confound the optimal balance of emotional distance and closeness between the doctor and the patient.[23] They regard these impulses as so significant a threat to physicians' abilities to respond objectively to patients' stated desires for death, as to be grounds for opposing the legalization of physician-assisted suicide. In support of his skepticism that legislative safeguards can prevent serious abuses of officially sanctioned physician aid-in-dying, Burt has recently written:

> Legalization of this practice also ostentatiously depends on the moral purity of all authorized actors: the dying person must be entirely free from tainted motives, from anything interfering with uncoerced choice; and those around the dying person (whether family or physician) must be equally pure and single-minded, without any self-interested wish to hasten that person's death. This is the breeding ground for unacknowledged abuse—for self-abuse by the dying person or abuse by others.[24]

Diane Meier and her colleagues have generalized the problem of the emotional impact on physicians of caring for seriously ill patients, beyond the specific dangers of participating in patients' suicides. They apply what they refer to as "the standard medical model of risk factors, signs and symptoms, differential diagnosis, and intervention" to a wide range of emotional responses that doctors might experience and the potential impact of their unexamined feelings on patient care.[25] With healthy-minded confidence in the power of a systematic approach, they recommend a five-step method for physicians to "respond constructively to the presence of the emotion": stepping back to gain perspective, identifying behaviors stemming from the feeling, considering implications and consequences, thinking through alternative outcomes of different behaviors, and consulting a trusted colleague.

While these prescriptions are undoubtedly beneficial to both doctor and patient, the sick soul views them as a thin container for the radioactive core of the doctor's existential moment—the intimation of chaos and disintegration that grasps us when we perceive ourselves to be on the threshold of death's dark kingdom. Jean Vanier, the Canadian pioneer in systems of support for people with severe developmental disabilities, expressed poetically the fear of our own undoing that can unhinge us when we are close to one who is about to die, or who otherwise bears the marks of life's great afflictions:

> and i am afraid . . .
> those haggard eyes
> or open wounds
> or black skin or white skin
> or alcoholic smell
> or freaked out mind
> of the man in misery
> strike deep chords of fear within me . . .
> fear of losing my money, time, reputation
> liberty.
> fear, above all, of losing myself
> fear of the unknown
> for misery is a world of the unknown . . .
> terror of despair,
> those hands . . . those hands . . .
> those hands stretched out towards
> me . . .

> *i am afraid to touch them . . .*
> *they may drag me down, down*
> *down to some unknown*
> *future . . .*
>
> *i fear my helplessness*
> *my hollows*
> *my poverty*
> *you remind me that i too must die*
> *. . .*
> *because i fear my emptiness*
> *my poverty*
> *my call to death*
> *i fear myself*
> *i close my heart . . . cement block . . .*
> *shut myself off*
> *from you,*
> *my despairing brother*[26]

Notwithstanding the virtues of physician introspection, communication skills training, stress reduction, burnout prevention, and other psychological coping mechanisms that are the common wisdom of enlightened end-of-life care, the sick soul cannot but wonder whether Vanier's evocation of existential dread in the presence of suffering and death may not, in James's words, "open a profounder view and put into our hands a more complicated key to the meaning of the situation." What might that meaning be, in the context of palliative care? What should we realistically expect from our increasing mastery of the physical, psychological, and social problems of the dying? One possible meaning is that the prospects for the fulfillment of our expectations are necessarily limited by the finitude of human ingenuity and stamina in the face of death's uncontainable power. That, while the current reforms in end-of-life care are certainly needed, we will be wise if we do not let our progress—slow as it is likely to be—make us forget what the theologian Dorothee Soelle suggested in the concluding words of her book, *Suffering*:

We can change the social conditions under which people experience suffering. We can change ourselves and learn in suffering instead of becoming worse. We can gradually beat back and abolish the suffering that is still produced for the profit of a few. But on all these paths we come up against boundaries that cannot be crossed. Death is not the only such barrier. There are also brutalization and insensibility, mutilation and injury that can no longer be reversed. The only way these boundaries can be crossed is by sharing the pain of the sufferers with them, not leaving them alone and making their cry louder.[27]

For Michael Kearney, Anne's final words to him suggested a similar meaning in the situation of the physician trying to do his or her best for one who is dying. Though Anne's words did not negate for him the importance of good palliative care or his own skills as a palliative care physician, they put them in a humbling perspective. "They are a reminder," Kearney wrote at the end of his narrative, "that despite all we might say and all we might do, the process of dying includes suffering and painful separations and unfinished business. Death cannot be tamed. Death is unknown. Death is other. Death is death."[28]

NOTES

1. Michael Kearney, *Mortally Wounded: Stories of Soul Pain, Death, and Healing* (New York: Scribner, 1996), 115–31.

2. Kearney, *Mortally Wounded*, 126–27.

3. Kearney, *Mortally Wounded*, 130.

4. In the acknowledgments of his book Kearney observes that caring for the dying is possible only through teamwork, and that "for editorial reasons what should sometimes read 'we' in the stories that follow has been simplified to 'I.'" It is impossible to tell whether his account of the decision to sedate Anne is one of those times. If Kearney did share the burden of this decision with his colleagues, this would of course alter somewhat the force of my comments. There is still no evidence, however, that Kearney attempted to determine Anne's own preference.

5. Michael Kearney, "Palliative Medicine—Just Another Specialty?" *Palliative Medicine* 6 (1992): 39–46.

6. Angela Fagerlin and Carl E. Schneider, "Enough: The Failure of the Living Will," *Hastings Center Report* 32, no. 2 (2004): 30–42.

7. National Hospice and Palliative Care Organization, *Facts and Figures* (Alexandria, Virginia, 2001).

8. Cynthia Pan, R. Sean Morrison, Diane Meier, D. K. Natale, S. L. Goldhirsch, P. Kralovec, and C. K. Cassel, "How Prevalent Are Hospital-Based Palliative Care Programs? Status Report and Future Directions," *Journal of Palliative Medicine* 4, no. 3 (fall 2001): 315–24.

9. Eric J. Cassell, "Dying in a Technological Society," in *Death Inside Out,* eds. Peter Steinfels and Robert M. Veatch (New York: Harper and Row, 1974), 48.

10. For the Robert Wood Johnson Foundation, see Ethan Bronner, "The Foundation's End-of-Life Programs: Changing the American Way of Death," in *To Improve Health Care, Volume VI, The Robert Wood Johnson Foundation Anthology,* eds. Stephen L. Isaacs and James R. Knickman (San Francisco: Jossey-Bass, 2003), 81–98. For the Project on Death in America, see Open Society Institute, *Transforming the Culture of Dying: The Project on Death in America, October 1994 to December 2003* (New York: Open Society Institute, 2004), 4.

11. Kathleen M. Foley and Hellen Gelband, eds., *Improving Palliative Care for Cancer* (Washington, D.C.: National Academy Press, 2001), 2.

12. Foley and Gelband, eds., *Improving Palliative Care for Cancer.*

13. Philippe Ariès, *The Hour of Our Death,* trans. Helen Weaver (New York: Oxford University Press, 1981), 610.

14. William James, *The Varieties of Religious Experience,* originally published in 1902 (London: Collins, 1960), 108.

15. James, *The Varieties of Religious Experience,* 102.

16. James, *The Varieties of Religious Experience,* 103.

17. James, *The Varieties of Religious Experience,* 103.

18. James, *The Varieties of Religious Experience,* 144–45.

19. James, *The Varieties of Religious Experience,* 149.

20. Leo Tolstoy, *The Death of Ivan Ilych,* trans. Aylmer Maude (New York: New American Library, 1960), 131–32.

21. Balfour M. Mount, "The Existential Moment," *Palliative and Supportive Care* 1 (2003): 93–96.

22. John Hinton, "The Dying and the Doctor," in *Man's Concern with Death,* ed. Arnold Toynbee (St. Louis: McGraw-Hill, 1969), 36.

23. Steven H. Miles, "Physicians and Their Patients' Suicides," *JAMA* 271 (1994): 1786–88; and Robert A. Burt, *Death Is That Man Taking Names: Intersections of American Medicine, Law, and Culture* (Berkeley: University of California Press, 2002).

24. Burt, *Death Is That Man Taking Names,* 163.

25. Diane E. Meier, Anthony L. Back, and R. Sean Morrison, "The Inner Life of Physicians and Care of the Seriously Ill," *JAMA* 286 (2001): 3007–14.

26. Jean Vanier, *Tears of Silence* (Toronto: Griffin House, 1970), 18–22. Quoted with permission from the publisher.

27. Dorothee Soelle, *Suffering* (Philadelphia: Fortress Press, 1975), 178.

28. Kearney, *Mortally Wounded,* 131.

5

Influence of Mental Illness on Decision Making at the End of Life

Linda Ganzini and Elizabeth R. Goy

In the United States, respect for autonomy is given great weight in clinical decision making. According to Beauchamp and Childress, autonomy is the "personal rule of the self that is free from both controlling interferences by others and from personal limitations that prevent meaningful choices, such as inadequate understanding."[1] In the medical context, respect for autonomy requires that clinicians allow patients to choose to forgo medical treatments, even if death results.[2]

Psychiatric disorders are the most common cause of loss of decision-making capacity in adults. Many individuals with a mental illness are autonomous and capable of self-determination; but others have varying degrees of impairment. Mental illness poses a threat to autonomy when it impairs decision-making abilities or renders individuals unable to act voluntarily.[3] In addition, patients who are institutionalized for their mental illness, or who are very dependent on others for basic needs, may lack the freedom to make decisions, even when they have sufficient cognitive abilities to weigh risks and benefits.[4] Finally, some psychiatric disorders are prevalent in terminally ill patients, including delirium, depression, and dementia.[5] But others, such as schizophrenia, substance abuse, or mania, are lifelong. They too can complicate decision making at the end of life.

In this chapter we consider how depression and schizophrenia can undermine autonomy in the terminally ill. We focus on these disorders because they are paradigmatic of how mental illness can complicate decision-making capacity assessment at the end of life. At times, clinicians err in assuming that the very presence of these illnesses automatically results in incompetence. This can lead them to fail to respect the legitimate decisions of these patients to refuse life-sustaining interventions. However, disorders associated with depression and schizophrenia are very heterogeneous and cause a range of severity of impairment. Consequently, assessment of decision-making capacity can be truly challenging to even experts in the field.

ASSESSING AUTONOMY

In the clinic, autonomy is assessed by reference to the patient's decision-making capacity or competence.[6] Grisso and Appelbaum identify four standards (or abilities) that are relevant to this assessment.[7] These include the ability of the patient (1) to express a choice, (2) to understand information relevant to his or her medical treatment, including risks, benefits, and alternatives, (3) to appreciate this information by applying it to his or her own personal situation, and (4) to make a rational decision, given his or her values and interests.[8]

Mental illness and incompetence are not synonymous.[9] Both schizophrenia and depression can impair decision making with respect to any one or all of the above standards. A great deal of thought and care is required on the part of the clinician to make a capacity determination. Although actual legal standards vary by jurisdiction, clinicians have *de facto*, if not *de jure,* authority to determine whether patients can make specific decisions and to identify surrogates for patients who lack decision-making ability.[10]

There is less agreement among experts regarding the thresholds used for each of the four standards. Many recommend a sliding scale, such that the higher the risks to the patient of refusal of treatment, the lower the threshold for declaring incompetence. For example, a clinician might require a higher level of understanding and appreciation for an otherwise healthy person to decline cardiopulmonary resuscitation than for a terminally ill patient to forgo the same procedure.[11] When a terminally ill patient declines a treatment of little value, the clinician will likely use a lenient threshold, rarely challenging the patient's thinking.[12] But some have expressed concern that the sliding scale leaves too much room for the clinician's values to usurp those of the patient, particularly if the physician raises the bar for patients who refuse interventions that the health care practitioner recommends.[13]

Clinicians' moral views on the sanctity of life or the importance of patient self-determination may influence their views on patients' competence to make decisions resulting in hastened death. We are not aware of studies that examine the effect of physicians' moral views on the standards they would use for competence to refuse life-sustaining treatment. However, in a study of standards for competence to pursue physician-assisted suicide (PAS), forensic psychiatrists who were morally opposed to PAS were more likely to advocate more stringent standards for competency evaluation. Fifty-eight percent of these experts believed, for example, that the diagnosis of depression should automatically result in a finding of incompetence.[14] Application of the above standards may help with this problem. Among experts in dementia, Marson et al. reported low levels of agreement about competence when examining patients with mild Alzheimer's disease.[15] However, when a common set of standards was applied by experts, their level of agreement improved.

In general, capacity evaluations are decision-specific; that is, patients may be able to make some decisions but not others.[16] For example, a patient with mild cognitive impairment may be unable to make a decision about chemotherapy that includes weighing trade-offs of modest survival benefits versus substantial short-term morbidity. The same patient might be able to complete a durable power of attorney for health care if she understands the surrogate's role and can identify whom she trusts to make decisions. At the end of life, evaluation of capacity for specific decisions can be simplified if the overall goals of care are ascertained. Although patients may wish that medical interventions benefit both survival and quality of life, they must often choose between these goals when in the final stages of their disease. For example, a patient with end-stage chronic obstructive pulmonary disease or cancer may prolong survival through ventilatory support in an intensive care unit, but at the cost of isolation, restrictions on mobility, pain, and agitated delirium. In contrast, a similarly ill patient who chooses hospice care forgoes most life-prolonging treatments. The focus of care in hospice is on symptom control in an environment, such as home, that minimizes restrictions and maximizes comfort. Once goals of care are determined for patients with advanced disease (with the poles being comfort/symptom control/palliation versus aggressive life-sustaining interventions), discussing and framing specific interventions, and assessing the consonance of specific decisions with goals becomes more straightforward.

REFUSING LIFE-SUSTAINING TREATMENTS

Legally, the patient's right to stop or never start life-sustaining treatments is grounded in the right of autonomous individuals to be free of unwanted, burdensome treatments.[17] In some situations patients may decline treatments, not because of objections to their burdens, but because they wish for death to come sooner. For competent patients, the legal legitimacy of the decision is not invalidated by the reason. Historically, however, clinicians have recognized that desire for hastened death may result from pathological psychological states. In patients with mental illness such as depression or schizophrenia, the decision to stop life-prolonging treatment may represent a suicidal equivalent that should, in some cases, be overridden by the health care team. Discerning whether decisions in mentally ill patients are autonomous can be very difficult. This is increasingly true, as forgoing life-prolonging treatment is gradually becoming the norm in terminally ill patients. In 70 percent of hospital deaths, a decision is made to withhold or withdraw some type of life-sustaining treatment.[18] Approximately 25 percent of all deaths in the United States occur in hospice.[19] Many hospice patients are competent and choose comfort, palliation, and quality of life over continued life-sustaining interventions. Among mentally ill patients with advanced disease there is the risk that if denied the right to refuse life-sustaining treatments, they are also deprived of the comfort and palliation that is increasingly the focus of care for other dying patients. Alternatively because aggressive life-sustaining care can be difficult to perform in mentally ill patients who resist, there is also the risk that clinicians too readily accede to the patients' decision to decline life-prolonging care.

DEPRESSION AND END-OF-LIFE DECISION MAKING

The primary feature of major depressive disorder is low mood or loss of pleasure in nearly all activities, most of the time, for at least two weeks. Other symptoms include disturbances in appetite, sleep and activity level; decreased energy; feelings of worthlessness or guilt; difficulty thinking or making decisions; and recurrent thoughts of death, suicidal ideation, plans or attempts.[20] Because the response to psychotherapy and pharmacotherapy in patients whose depression is "reactive" to a stressful life event is no better or worse than response in an "endogenous" depression that has intermittently occurred throughout life, these distinctions are no longer made.[21] The diagnosis of depression is complicated in physically ill patients as clinicians are often uncertain whether to attribute somatic symptoms such as weight loss and fatigue to depression or medical illness. Chochinov et al. reported that when psychological symptoms are at least moderately severe, somatic items cease to contribute substantially to diagnostic variance.[22] That is, it is less important how much weight loss or fatigue a person has than how severe the anhedonia or low mood is. Using these more stringent criteria, approximately 10 percent of terminally ill patients meet criteria for major depressive disorder.[23]

Concerns regarding mental illness as a potentially treatable cause of patients' refusal of life-sustaining treatment stem from the known relationship between depression and suicide. Among both physically ill and healthy persons, depression is powerfully associated with suicidal ideations, suicide attempts, and completed suicide. Experts on suicide prevention and depression treatment strongly encourage clinicians to treat depression aggressively and do what is needed to avert suicide. Suicide prevention is effective though patients remain at risk, especially among the elderly. For example, Hepple and Quinton reported on one hundred consecutive referrals for suicidal ideation in persons over age sixty-five years. At follow-up, ranging from two to five years, forty-two patients had died, twelve of suicide.[24] In examining the seven-year outcome of 137 patients who presented for suicidality in Texas, twelve ultimately died of suicide.[25] These studies support that suicide prevention averts 85 percent to 90 percent of suicides, but also that depression portends nonsuicidal deaths in older persons.

Depression treatment is effective—only 29 percent to 46 percent of depressed patients have little or no response to antidepressants.[26] After successful treatment of depression in community and primary care populations, the reported rates of recurrence are low, ranging from 30 percent to 40 percent.[27] There are no randomized, controlled trials of depression treatment in terminally ill patients, however. Antidepressants are effective after several weeks, leaving little time to respond among patients at the end of life. The long-term outcome of late-life depression among psychiatric patients is poor. For example, among 277 depressed Dutch patients followed for six years, only 23 percent had a full remission.[28] Studies from the United Kingdom demonstrate high rates of nonsuicidal death among depressed elderly patients. Only 22 percent to 33 percent of survivors experience full remissions from the mood disorder.[29]

Hopelessness is an even stronger predictor of suicidal ideation than is depression.[30] Hopelessness is a way of thinking in which negative expectations about the future are pervasive. Depressed patients may develop hopelessness as they begin to doubt that they will ever improve or enjoy life again. Hopeless patients endorse that the future looks dark to them and they are convinced that there will be no opportunities for improvement.[31] Hopelessness can occur as a manifestation of depression, but also an independent perception.

Among patients with advanced medical illness, studies support that depression and hopelessness are strong and consistent risk factors for endorsing that they want death to come sooner.[32] For example, in a study of two hundred terminally ill patients with cancer in a palliative care hospital, desire for hastened death was associated with both depression and hopelessness, each of which provided independent and unique contributions to the patients who hope that death would come sooner.[33] Chochinov et al. reported that of 168 palliative care patients depression predicted failing will to live.[34] Among two hundred Canadian cancer palliative care patients, major depressive disorder was the factor most strongly associated with desire for hastened death.[35] This very strong relationship between depression, hopelessness, desire for hastened death and suicide has naturally led to the concern that decisions to stop life-sustaining treatment reflect depression. Instead of respecting the decision, the clinician should redouble efforts to diagnose and aggressively treat the depression, all the while protecting the patient from their self-murderous impulses.

Theoretically, depression could impair decision making with respect to several of the standards outlined by Grisso and Appelbaum.[36] Depression might cause ambivalence or such apathy that patients cannot or will not express a choice. Severely depressed patients can develop cognitive impairment such that they cannot evaluate the risks and benefits of a treatment. Hopelessness most often impacts the ability to appreciate the information. A hopeless worldview can temporarily alter one's formula for weighing risks and benefits, leading the patient to undervalue good outcomes or focus excessively on risks or the difficulty of tolerating the burdens of treatment. When patients decide to forgo treatment, we hope that the decision reflects an underlying set of stable values or a life philosophy. Depression may alter values temporarily, so that decisions no longer reflect the authentic self.

Yet studies of the association between depression and refusal of treatment do not yield consistent results. Using hypothetical scenarios of illness, Lee and Ganzini found that mild to moderate depression had a small association with preferences toward life-sustaining medical treatment in older patients hospitalized on medical units.[37] An association was only found in scenarios with good prognosis, but not poor prognosis. All study participants were referred for depression treatment. At follow-up, there was no consistent increase in preference for life-prolonging therapy associated with depression resolution. Compared to those in the never depressed group, the depressed patients were more inconsistent in their preferences when examined longitudinally, suggesting the need to repeat advanced care planning and reassess preferences over time.[38]

Blank et al. reported similar results when comparing seventy-one depressed patients from a general medical hospital to eighty-one nondepressed patients. The two groups did not differ in level of desire for treatments when examining several scenarios, including a terminal condition. When financial impact was introduced, however, significantly more depressed subjects refused treatment options that they had previously wanted compared to nondepressed subjects. Passive suicidality (a desire to die in the absence of a plan to suicide), was strongly predictive of life-sustaining treatment refusal.[39] Cohen et al. prospectively studied patients who discontinued dialysis.[40] Among twenty-three patients who stopped this life-sustaining treatment, the prevalence of major depression was only 10 percent. This proportion is similar to the prevalence of depression in physically ill patients overall.

In contrast, of 1,590 patients analyzed in the SUPPORT study, greater depression was associated with a change over two months to preferring do-not-resuscitate (DNR) status. For patients initially preferring DNR, those with substantial improvements in depression scores between interviews were more than five times as likely to change preference to want CPR than were patients with substantial worsening in depression score.[41]

Studies that examine depressed psychiatric inpatients show somewhat different results, likely reflecting greater severity in mood disorders. Among forty-three depressed, elderly psychiatric inpatients, an increase in desire for life-sustaining medical therapy occurred after depression treatment in those who were initially rated as more depressed, more hopeless, and more likely to overestimate the risks and underestimate the benefits of treatment. The data support that when depression influences choices it is not occult, but obvious to a skilled clinician.[42] Similarly, Lifton and Kettl reviewed the medical records of 191 geriatric psychiatric inpatients with major depressive disorder or bipolar disorder.[43] Patients with suicidal ideation were significantly more likely to prefer DNR status.

Overall, these studies suggest depression of mild to moderate severity does not impair decision-making capacity, although the preferences of patients with this kind of depression may be more variable over time. Clinicians may need to explore mildly depressed patients' reasoning in documented discussions more frequently. Among patients with moderate to severe depression or who are ill enough to be admitted to a psychiatric facility, new advance care planning should be deferred. Depressed and psychologically suffering patients can infect their providers with hopelessness such that clinicians fail to see the treatable aspects. Depression is not a natural or inevitable part of terminal illness and such views should not influence assessments on the treatability of mood disorders. In the case of very psychiatrically ill patients who wish to stop life-sustaining treatment, family should be engaged to help determine if decisions are congruent with values and preferences expressed and decisions made when not depressed. Clearly written directives executed when not depressed should be honored. On the other hand, a decision to refuse a life-sustaining treatment such as CPR should not be overruled automatically since such interventions are commonly refused by nondepressed patients. Severe depression with advanced physical illness has a poor prognosis. Depression compounds suffering in terminally ill patients. If mandatory life-sustaining treatment for depressed patients was imposed through concern that their preference may change, many comfortable deaths would be denied.

DECISION MAKING FOR PATIENTS WITH SCHIZOPHRENIA AT THE END OF LIFE

Schizophrenia is an illness that afflicts approximately 1 percent of the population.[44] This disorder often results in grave and progressive disability with social and occupational dysfunction. Patients with schizophrenia suffer from delusions—often paranoid—hallucinations, disorganized thinking, and odd behaviors. Negative symptoms compound interpersonal difficulties—patients often have poor eye contact, restricted or inappropriate expressions of emotion, impoverished speech, apathy, and difficulties initiating and persisting with goal-directed activities.[45] Patients with schizophrenia often have cognitive impairment, especially in the frontal lobe processes that allow mental flexibility and abstraction—all abilities important to decision making that result in lack of insight or even denial of the existence of psychiatric and medical illnesses. These factors may impact physician-patient communication and impede development of rapport and a working alliance. There is little research about the care that patients with schizophrenia receive at the end of life or how decisions are made. However, a review of what is known about treatment of medical problems in patients with schizophrenia and their decisional abilities can inform this discussion.

In general, patients with psychosis receive suboptimal medical care. Patient-related reasons include lack of financial resources, lack of skills to use the health care system appropriately, lack of adherence to treatment, difficulty keeping appointments or sitting in waiting rooms, difficulty reporting symptoms accurately, and refusal of recommendations. About one-third of patients with schizophrenia do not believe that they have a mental illness.[46] Studies of patients' acknowledgement of their medical diagnoses are not available, but case reports suggest similar disavowal of physical illness and terminal illness.[47]

Many psychotic patients fail to adhere to medical and psychiatric treatments. For example, only 40 percent of veteran patients with schizophrenia adhere to recommended antipsychotic treatment, even though the VA provides medication at no cost.[48] Veterans with psychotic disorders were found to be similarly nonadherent with antihypertensives, antihyperlipidemics, and antidiabetics.[49] Lack of adherence or insight result in patients presenting with more advanced disease. Older schizophrenic patients report fewer physical illnesses, but these tended to be more severe. Patients who present with very advanced states of cancer, for example, unusual fungating and ulcerating cancerous skin lesions, often have a comorbid diagnosis of schizophrenia and often require involuntary treatment of their medical illness. Some authors report that schizophrenic patients are less likely to report pain or discomfort with acute illness, including myocardial infarctions, burns, perforated peptic ulcers, and gangrenous extremities.[50] For primary care physicians, these difficulties may result in need for increased time and coordination with mental health practitioners to provide care.

Schizophrenia can be associated with impairments in decision-making capacity impacting abilities in any of the standards outlined by Grisso and Appelbaum.[51] For example, extreme ambivalence can render individuals with schizophrenia unable to make a stable decision. Patients may be unable to appreciate their choices if they deny that they have a terminal disease. Frontal lobe impairments may result in limited abstractional abilities necessary to weigh risk and benefits, while delusions or hallucinations may result in irrational thought processes relevant to acceptance of treatment.

Approximately half of patients with schizophrenia have impairments in decision-making abilities; they are more impaired than depressed and nonmentally ill groups, although there is considerable heterogeneity among patients. In a study by Grisso and Appelbaum, patients with high levels of thought disorder and delusions were particularly at risk of incompetence.[52] In contrast, studies of ability to consent to research suggest that cognitive impairment results in difficulties understanding consent forms. These disabilities can be overcome with enhanced informed consent procedures such as educational videotapes and repetition of pertinent concepts. Improvement in decision-making ability is such that after these interventions, there were no differences between patients with schizophrenia and nonmentally ill controls.[53] These enhanced procedures serve as a model for discussion with health care providers about treatment choices. Despite the high proportion of patients with denial of illness, several recent studies report that patients with schizophrenia describe low satisfaction with the amount of information they receive regarding their care; that they want to be actively involved in their health care decisions, yet perceive that participation is limited.[54]

Information is lacking on several aspects of decision making for patients with schizophrenia at the end of life. It is unclear how decisions regarding course of care are made, who makes the decisions, and how often care must be administered under coercive settings. It is unknown how informed schizophrenic patients are regarding their terminal diagnoses, the nature of the conversations about their terminal illness, how mental health and medical clinicians work together around these issues, and what the special needs of patients with schizophrenia in palliative and hospice care are.

Despite their vulnerabilities patients with schizophrenia should be told about a life-threatening diagnosis. Many patients may, with repetition, and review of relevant information, be able to understand the decisions to be made. Others will maintain a strong denial of their diagnosis, its severity, and needs for treatment. Efforts should be made to continue to work to explain the diagnosis and decisions, with careful monitoring to make sure that the psychosis does not worsen in the attempt. Some patients will have had a lifelong difficulty with such decisions and defer to family members or their mental health providers. As with other patients, they can assign decision making to others. Surrogate decision-makers should be found for patients who fail to accept their illness, have too much cognitive impairment, or are too disorganized to manage.

Lack of decision-making capacity because of denial of illness should not mandate life-sustaining treatment. Patients treated against their will cannot be comforted by knowing their immediate suffering has reason or purpose. Coercive settings and treatments to prolong life should occur only when there is a high likelihood of improved survival or clear opportunities for amelioration of suffering. It is possible that patients with schizophrenia may find hospice and palliative care as objectionable as life-sustaining treatment. Isolative and paranoid patients may find personal care and the emphasis on closure and relationships that are the focus of hospice care, threatening and overwhelming.[55]

MENTAL HEALTH CONSULTATION

Mental health consultation can be useful in evaluating the competence and authenticity of decision making for patients with severe depression and schizophrenia who wish to refuse life-sustaining treatment. Several caveats, however, are important to keep in mind. The primary responsibility for determining competence to consent or to refuse treatment always remains with the primary treating clinician. Primary care clinicians have several advantages in assessing competence—they may know the patient and understand the treatments better than the mental health clinician. Mental health training does not result in immunity from having moral concerns influencing assessments. Psychiatrists and psychologists, however, are more familiar with how psychosis and depression influence thinking. Additionally, they are best able to treat these disorders, which if successful, may result in recovery of decision-making abilities.[56]

NOTES

1. T. L. Beauchamp and J. F. Childress, *Principles of Biomedical Ethics*, 4th ed. (New York: Oxford University Press, 1994), 121.

2. L. Ganzini, I. Volicer, W. A. Nelson, et al., "Ten Myths About Decision-Making Capacity," *Journal of the American Medical Directors Association* 5 (2004): 263–67.

3. B. Lo, *Resolving Ethical Dilemmas: A Guide for Clinicians* (Baltimore, Md.: Williams & Wilkins, 1995).

4. L. W. Roberts, "Informed Consent and the Capacity for Voluntarism," *American Journal of Psychiatry* 159 (2002): 705–12.

5. E. R. Goy and L. Ganzini, "Delirium, Anxiety, and Depression," in *Geriatric Palliative Care*, eds. R. S. Morrison, D. E. Meier, and C. Capello (Oxford: Oxford University Press, 2003).

6. Many authors distinguish between "decision-making capacity" as assessed by clinicians and "competence" as determined by a court. Grisso and Appelbaum make the case for using the term "competence" to indicate a state in which decision-

making capacities are sufficient enough to be honored, regardless of who makes the decision. We use these terms interchangeably in this chapter to indicate clinician assessed capacities.

7. T. Grisso and P. S. Appelbaum, *Assessing Competence to Consent to Treatment: A Guide for Physicians and Other Health Professionals* (New York: Oxford University Press, 1998).

8. Grisso and Appelbaum, *Assessing Competence to Consent to Treatment*, 58.

9. Grisso and Appelbaum, *Assessing Competence to Consent to Treatment*.

10. Ganzini, Volicer, and Nelson, et al. "Ten Myths About Decision-Making Capacity."

11. L. Ganzini, I. Volicer, W. A. Nelson, et al., "Pitfalls in Assessment of Decision-Making Capacity." *Psychosomatics* 44 (2003): 237–43.

12. M. D. Sullivan, L. Ganzini, and S. Youngner, "Should Psychiatrists Serve as Gatekeepers for Physician-Assisted Suicide?" *Hastings Center Report* 28 (1998): 24–31.

13. Ganzini, Volicer, Nelson, et al., "Pitfalls in Assessment of Decision-Making Capacity." In a survey of almost four hundred psychiatrists, psychologists, and geriatricians on their views about the most common pitfalls in assessing patient decision-making capacity, 90 percent of respondents agreed that "not understanding that criteria for determining capacity to make a decision vary with the risks and benefits inherent in the decision" was an important error. See cite note 11.

14. L. Ganzini, G. B. Leong, D. S. Fenn, et al., "Evaluation of Competence to Consent to Assisted Suicide: Views of Forensic Psychiatrists," *American Journal of Psychiatry* 157 (2000): 595–600.

15. D. C. Marson, K. S. Earnst, F. Jamil, et al., "Consistency of Physicians' Legal Standard and Personal Judgments of Competency in Patients with Alzheimer's Disease," *JAGS* 48 (2000): 911–18.

16. Grisso and Appelbaum, *Assessing Competence to Consent to Treatment*.

17. Lo, *Resolving Ethical Dilemmas: A Guide for Clinicians*.

18. M. J. Field and C. K. Cassel, *Approaching Death: Improving Care at the End of Life* (Washington, D.C.: National Academy Press, 1997).

19. National Hospice and Palliative Care Organization, *Facts and Figures on Hospice Care in America* (Alexandria, Va.: National Hospice and Palliative Care Organization, 2003).

20. American Psychiatric Association, *Diagnostic and Statistical Manual of Mental Disorders: DSM-IV.*, 4th ed. (Washington, D.C.: American Psychiatric Association, 1994.)

21. L. Ganzini, "Commentary: Assessment of Clinical Depression in Patients Who Request Physician-Assisted Death," *Journal of Pain and Symptom Management* 19 (2000): 474–78.

22. H. M. Chochinov, K. G. Wilson, M. Enns, et al., "Prevalence of Depression in the Terminally Ill: Effects of Diagnostic Criteria and Symptom Threshold Judgments," *American Journal of Psychiatry* 151 (1994): 537–40.

23. Chochinov, Wilson, Enns, et al., "Prevalence of Depression in the Terminally Ill."

24. J. Hepple and C. Quinton, "One Hundred Cases of Attempted Suicide in the Elderly," *British Journal of Psychiatry* 171 (1997): 42–46.

25. M. T. Lambert, "Seven-Year Outcomes of Patients Evaluated for Suicidality," *Psychiatric Services* 53 (2002): 92–94.

26. M. Fava and K. G. Davidson, "Definition and Epidemiology of Treatment-Resistant Depression," *Psychiatric Clinics of North America* 19 (1996): 179–200.

27. E. M. van Weel-Baumgarten, H. J. Schers, W. J. van den Bosch, et al., "Long-Term Follow-Up of Depression among Patients in the Community and in Family Practice Settings: A Systematic Review," *Journal of Family Practice* 49 (2000): 1113–20.

28. A. T. Beekman, S. W. Geerlings, D. J. Deeg, et al., "The Natural History of Late-Life Depression: A Six-Year Prospective Study in the Community," *Archives of General Psychiatry* 59 (2002): 605–11.

29. V. K. Sharma, J. R. Copeland, M. E. Dewey, et al., "Outcome of the Depressed Elderly Living in the Community in Liverpool: A Five-Year Follow-Up," *Psychological Medicine* 28 (1998): 1329–37. See also G. Livingston, V. Watkin, B. Milne, et al., "The Natural History of Depression and the Anxiety Disorders in Older People: The Islington Community Study," *Journal of Affective Disorders* 46 (1997): 255–62.

30. H. M. Chochinov, K. G. Wilson, M. Enns, et al., "Depression, Hopelessness, and Suicidal Ideation in the Terminally Ill," *Psychosomatics* 39 (1998): 366–70.

31. A. T. Beck, A. Lester, et al., "The Measurement of Pessimism: The Hopelessness Scale," *Journal of Consulting and Clinical Psychology* 42 (1974): 861–65.

32. E. J. Emanuel, D. L. Fairclough, and L. L. Emanuel, "Attitudes and Desires Related to Euthanasia and Physician-Assisted Suicide among Terminally Ill Patients and Their Caregivers," *JAMA* 284 (2000): 2460–68. See also K. G. Wilson, J. F. Scott, I. D. Graham, et al., "Attitudes of Terminally Ill Patients toward Euthanasia and Physician-Assisted Suicide," *Archives of Internal Medicine* 160 (2000): 2454–60. T. Akechi, H. Okamura, and S. Yamawaki, et al., "Why Do Some Cancer Patients with Depression Desire an Early Death and Others Do Not?" *Psychosomatics* 42 (2001): 141–45. M. Lloyd-Williams, "How Common Are Thoughts of Self-Harm in a UK Palliative Care Population?" *Supportive Care Cancer* 10 (2002): 422–24.

33. W. Breitbart, B. Rosenfeld, and H. Pessin, et al., "Depression, Hopelessness, and Desire for Hastened Death in Terminally Ill Patients with Cancer," *JAMA* 284 (2000): 2907–11.

34. H. M. Chochinov, D. Tataryn, J. J. Clinch, et al., "Will to Live in the Terminally Ill," *Lancet* 354 (1999): 816–19.

35. H. M. Chochinov, K. G. Wilson, and M. Enns, et al., "Desire for Death in the Terminally Ill," *American Journal of Psychiatry* 152, no. 8 (1995): 1185–91.

36. Grisso and Appelbaum, *Assessing Competence to Consent to Treatment.*

37. M. A. Lee and L. Ganzini, "Depression in the Elderly: Effect on Patient Attitudes toward Life-Sustaining Therapy," *Journal of the American Geriatrics Society* 40 (1992): 983–88.

38. M. A. Lee and L. Ganzini, "The Effect of Recovery from Depression on Preferences for Life-Sustaining Therapy in Older Patients," *The Journal of Gerontology* 49 (1994): M15–M21.

39. K. Blank, J. Robison, E. Doherty, et al., "Life-Sustaining Treatment and Assisted Death Choices in Depressed Older Patients," *Journal of the American Geriatrics Society* 49 (2001): 153–61.

40. L. M. Cohen, S. K. Dobscha, K. C. Hails, et al., "Depression and Suicidal Ideation in Patients Who Discontinue the Life-Support Treatment of Dialysis," *Psychosomatic Medicine* 64 (2002): 889–96.

41. K. E. Rosenfeld, N. S. Wenger, R. S. Phillips, et al., "Factors Associated with Change in Resuscitation Preference of Seriously Ill Patients: The SUPPORT Investigators Study to Understand Prognoses and Preferences for Outcomes and Risks of Treatments," *Archives of Internal Medicine* 156 (1996): 1558–64.

42. L. Ganzini, M. A. Lee, R. T. Heintz, et al., "The Effect of Depression Treatment on Elderly Patients' Preferences for Life-Sustaining Medical Therapy," *American Journal of Psychiatry* 151 (1994): 1631–36.

43. I. Lifton and P. A. Kettl, "Suicidal Ideation and the Choice of Advance Directives By Elderly Persons with Affective Disorders," *Psychiatric Services* 51 (2000): 1447–49.

44. American Psychiatric Association, *Diagnostic and Statistical Manual of Mental Disorders.*

45. American Psychiatric Association, *Diagnostic and Statistical Manual of Mental Disorders.*

46. J. M. Pyne, D. Bean, and G. Sullivan, "Characteristics of Patients with Schizophrenia Who Do Not Believe They Are Mentally Ill," *Journal of Nervous & Mental Disease* 189 (2001): 146–53.

47. Pyne, Bean, and Sullivan, "Characteristics of Patients with Schizophrenia Who Do Not Believe They Are Mentally Ill." See also T. L. Irvin, "Legal, Ethical and Clinical Implications of Prescribing Involuntary Life-Threatening Treatment: The Case of the Sunshine Kid," *Journal of Forensic Science* 48 (2003): 856–60; and M. J. Craun, M. Watkins, A. Hefty, "Hospice Care of the Psychotic Patient," *American Journal of Hospice and Palliative Care* 14 (1997): 205–8.

48. M. Valenstein, F. C. Blow, L. A. Copeland, et al., "Poor Antipsychotic Adherence among Patients with Schizophrenic Medication and Patient Factors," *Schizophrenia Bulletin* 30 (2004): 255–64.

49. C. R. Dolder, J. P. Lacro, and D. V. Jeste, "Adherence to Antipsychotic and Nonpsychiatric Medications in Middle-Aged and Older Patients with Psychotic Disorders," *Psychosomatic Medicine* 65 (2003): 156–62.

50. Craun, Watkins, Hefty, "Hospice Care of the Psychotic Patient." See also J. A. Talbott and L. Linn, "Reactions of Schizophrenics to Life-Threatening Dis-

ease," *Psychiatric Quarterly* 50 (1978): 218–27; and D. Goldenberg, J. Holland, and S. Schachter, "Palliative Care in the Chronically Mentally Ill," in *Handbook of Psychiatry in Palliative Medicine*, eds. H. M. Chochinov and W. Breitbart (Oxford: Oxford University Press, 2000).

51. Grisso and Appelbaum, *Assessing Competence to Consent to Treatment*.

52. T. Grisso and P. S. Appelbaum, "The MacArthur Treatment Competence Study III: Abilities of Patients to Consent to Psychiatric and Medical Treatments," *Law and Human Behavior* 19 (1995): 149–74.

53. L. B. Dunn and D. V. Jeste, "Problem Areas in the Understanding of Informed Consent for Research: Study of Middle-Aged and Older Patients with Psychotic Disorders," *Psychopharmacology* 171 (2003): 81–85. See also P. G. Stiles, N. G. Poythress, A. Hall, et al., "Improving Understanding of Research Consent Disclosures among Persons with Mental Illness," *Psychiatric Services* 52 (2001): 780–85; and W. T. J. Carpenter, J. M. Gold, A. C. Lahti, et al., "Decisional Capacity for Informed Consent in Schizophrenia Research," *Archives of General Psychiatry* 57 (2000): 533–38.

54. M. Ruggeri, A. Lasalvia, G. Bisoffi, et al., "Satisfaction with Mental Health Services among People with Schizophrenia in Five European Sites: Results from the EPSILON Study," *Schizophrenia Bulletin* 29 (2003): 229–45. See also R. Tempier, "Long-Term Psychiatric Patients' Knowledge about Their Medication," *Psychiatric Services* 47 (1996): 1385–87.

55. Craun, Watkins, Hefty, "Hospice Care of the Psychotic Patient."

56. Ganzini, Volicer, Nelson, et al., "Pitfalls in Assessment of Decision-Making Capacity." See also Ganzini, Volicer, Nelson, et al., "Ten Myths About Decision-Making Capacity."

6

Creative Adaptation in Aging and Dying: Ethical Imperative or Impossible Dream?

Celia Berdes and Linda Emanuel

How to treat the elderly and the dying is a core issue for every society. The central place held by the issue is evidenced by the fact that every major cultural and religious tradition sets out precepts to guide its members on how to behave toward their elderly and their dying. Though ever present, such precepts are also constantly evolving, and the questions raised thereby seem newly perplexing and urgent for each culture and each generation.

It is likewise well known that the post–World War II period spawned a population boom generation, the members of which will soon begin to cross into old age. In that period, biotechnical advances brought the promise of extended life and, some would argue, the mirage of indefinitely postponed death. Others have argued that this mirage was complicit in the creation of a dominant "youth culture" that embraced vitality and independence and eschewed age and interdependence. Whether or not the "baby boomers" will live longer than their elders, having been the embodiment of the youth culture, they aspire to an unprecedented level of vitality in old age. They are prepared to go to unprecedented lengths to meet the "vital aging" imperative—by improving their health behaviors, by "investing" in plastic surgery, and by spending discretionary funds on medical procedures. However, the boomers now face the flip side of the promises of biotechnology. In addition to or instead of the healthy continuation of middle age they envision, they are beginning to face a heavy burden of chronic disease and functional impairment. They are also confronted by the crushing reality that our economy likely cannot afford the expensive support systems necessary to sustain their quality of life.[1] Moreover, as Lloyd[2] has recently pointed out, because increasing proportions of people are living long lives, old age and death and dying are increasingly overlapping issues. This overlap sits uncomfortably for those who adhere to the "vital aging" paradigm. So today these questions remain more pressing than ever: How are we to age well? How are we to die well? How are we to care well for the aging and dying?

This chapter first considers what contemporary society should do in view of the fact that aging and dying have become extended components of the life cycle. We argue that this new reality requires that individuals and society more generally develop goals for care of the elderly and dying that are both realistic and ethical. We also argue for development of related, equally realistic and ethical goals for research and policy concerning services for those in these last stages of the life cycle. We identify five general aims toward that end, three that apply to individual situations and two that apply to communities or populations: (1) to understand and use the variety of individually-identified, life cycle-appropriate goals for care; (2) to use systematic comprehensive patient assessment to identify needs in a consistent way; (3) to foster a new paradigm of creative adaptation by individuals; (4) to make use of comprehensive population assessment, thus providing information to guide both research and policy about services; and finally (5) to make use of all these approaches within a context that expects elders to assume life cycle-related, dignified roles in society. The chapter goes on in a sixth section to consider a specific feature of aging that seems especially challenging, namely dementia. Using dementia as an exemplar, it considers how the imperatives identified in the first section should guide dementia care and dementia research toward finding realistic and ethical responses in the current era. In a concluding section, the chapter considers the social setting of aging and possibilities for the aforementioned realistic and ethical responses to these identified challenges.

AGING AND DYING AS LIFE CYCLE STAGES:
IMPLICATIONS FOR GOALS OF CARE

Aging has long been acknowledged as a stage of the life cycle, with its own age-appropriate tasks and social roles. Even so, our language lacks an equivalent term to that used for children or adults—childhood or adulthood—for the old age stage of the life cycle. Terms such as "elders" and descriptors such as "sage" and "wise" for older adults do exist, but there is no term for "oldhood."

It is even less firmly established that dying brings with it many tasks—some similar to those of "oldhood"—and social roles, independent of the dying person's age. Dying people, if they are given sufficient time, usually seek to close their life stories with as positive an ending as possible. If they can, they engage the "tasks of dying." They seek to leave their practical affairs in order and make arrangements so that those they care about will benefit from their material possessions. As well, they seek to pass on their roles to those they trust and care for, and they seek to lodge their life stories with someone who will remember and weave it into the future. In so doing, they take on the dying role, becoming at the same time dependent and omnipotent; those around them take on the role of carers and "heirs" to the mantles they expect to receive.[3]

Some of these tasks of dying are affected by the age of the dying person. Some are made easier by advanced age. For the elderly, much life has been lived and the care of young dependents is not often a source of anxiety.[4] On the other hand, many ordinary tasks of dying are magnified by old age. As the losses of illness and age multiply—with their attendant physical disabilities, mental capacity losses, and declines in social capital as friends and relatives also become ill and die—the capacity for adaptation becomes harder to muster. Circumstances and anxieties about the future also differ. Becoming dependent after a lifetime of independence can be difficult. Isolation, insolvency, and loss of cognitive ability become looming fears.[5]

Some older people respond to these realities by finding life a state not much better than death.[6] Others find that whatever life is left to them, even in the presence of profound losses, becomes all the more precious.[7] Generalizations about the aged dying are thus of only modest help for the clinician or care provider. It is fair and helpful to start with the expectation that many elders will have goals for their care that relate to their "oldhood" tasks and roles, and if applicable, to their conception of their dying tasks and roles. But still, the compelling need is to recognize that highly varied subjective experiences of life exist and therefore diverse goals for care exist.[8] The clinician must inquire and, if necessary, help the patient discern her own goals for care.

Goals for Care

Goals for care can range from wanting intervention for any and all ailments (with the aim of cure if possible and maximum delay in the illness' consequences if cure is impossible and with no limits placed on invasiveness or expense or other burden) to wanting comfort care only (with the aim of letting the illness run its natural course or prioritizing comfort over longevity). Often, goals fall somewhere between the two, or more likely entail a set of treatments that have a mixture of curative and palliative intent. The existence of various coexisting and equally legitimate goals obliges the clinician to inquire of patients how they see their life options and consequent goals for care and then to offer what help the clinician can in informing the individual's understanding and choices, in tailoring the individual's care to those choices, and thereby optimizing the outcomes of their care.[9]

This simple yet critically important notion of ascertaining life goals and using those goals as guides to orchestrate goals for care is—surprisingly—not central to traditional forms of care for the elderly and dying. The notion dropped away from modern medicine in the face of the unspoken assumption—fed by biotechnical advances in the postwar period that in turn fed inflated hopes of cure—that the paramount goal should be to cure disease. However, ancient medical declarations such as the Hippocratic oath are clear in assuming that much of medicine has to be oriented toward the patient's comfort and dignity.[10] The notion of goals for care has been promoted again more recently by the end-of-life care movement, and through the influence of that movement, is receiving new consideration across the field of medicine, including in geriatrics and palliative care, and in society at large.[11] The health care community in all its constituencies should acknowledge and seek ways to institutionalize the notion that patients' goals should guide goals of care, and that the two overarching goals, cure and comfort, can be harnessed together in that effort.

COMPREHENSIVE ASSESSMENT: A CORNERSTONE OF GOOD CARE

Although the explicit step of discerning goals for care has not been central in geriatrics practice, a corollary process—the comprehensive assessment—has been a central "clarion call" as the field of geriatrics has established its standing as a specialty discipline within medicine. By definition, the comprehensive assessment includes information about the history of physical and mental illnesses and the physical examination. It also pursues a much fuller than traditional inquiry into the social circumstances of the patient. The comprehensive assessment has been promoted on the same grounds as goals for care: without a full understanding of the patient, it is not possible to design or implement an optimal plan of care (Camann and Chase, 2001.)[12] Yet, in too many venues, comprehensive assessment has been seen as "Cadillac care," available only to those who can pay privately or those in special circumstances of need. To the contrary, clinicians should seize on and promote comprehensive assessment and goals-driven decision making as the essence of good care.

The palliative care movement has brought its own version of comprehensive assessment (known more often as "whole-patient assessment" in palliative care), and in so doing has allowed a helpful compare-and-contrast with that developed within geriatrics. The key difference is that the palliative care version includes more attention to the spiritual dimension of illness experience than the geriatrics version. To the extent that illness is experienced in the spiritual dimension and to the extent that spiritual life can provide a helpful coping mechanism and sometimes a helpful social setting that reduces the burdens of illness, this inclusion is helpful and should be further adopted in the geriatrics community.

Often, it is the case that patients and their families do not have a clear sense of their own goals for care. Part of the importance of comprehensive assessment is that it affords not only the clinicians but also the patient and family a chance to take a global look at their situation and discern what are the fitting, i.e., most realistic and best, goals for care available to them. Comprehensive assessment can be seen as preventive medicine in that it preempts needless, costly, and suffering-associated attempts to provide interventions that do not suit the goals of care that the patient wants or can realistically seek.

The comprehensive assessment or whole-patient assessment should not be limited to the very old or the obviously dying patient. The palliative care movement has reframed its scope more broadly to include palliative care as it applies to all patients, whether terminally ill or not, who need symptom management and a whole person focus. This reframing implies that what have hitherto been end-of-life care techniques will move "upstream" in the course of care, to begin at a point in time much closer to the time of diagnosis, and will become part of the forms of care patients already receive, such as long-term care. In this way, palliative care will become an integral part of comprehensive care for all patients, including but not limited to geriatrics. With this new orientation, comprehensive assessment and the use of goals of care will become an integral part of all geriatric care.

CREATIVE ADAPTATION: A STRATEGY
FOR ADAPTIVE AGING

A common feature of old age and dying is that desired outcomes simply are not available. The older person and the terminally ill person face progressively accruing losses: loss of exercise capacity, mental capacity, functions of daily living, social roles, and loved ones, to name a few. A key to attaining a sense of wholeness and fulfillment even in the face of inevitable major losses is the ability to adapt to these losses.

Hence, the issue of how elders can adapt to the challenge of serious illness must also be recognized and dealt with. The full range of supportive care options is not available and accessible to many elders; other elders may lack the capacity or social support to pursue a full range of care options that are otherwise within their grasp. Suboptimal or even maladaptive approaches to coping may yield suboptimal goals selected by the patient; then, the risk is that a simplistic deference to autonomy by care providers will bypass the possibility of fostering a more creative approach to adaptation by the patient and the development of better goals that the patient can adopt.

We would propose the concept and practice of creative adaptation as a coordinated response by the elder and his or her caregivers, both formal and informal. What is creative adaptation? Perhaps an initial definition must state what it is not: It is not successful aging, as it was defined by projects associated with the MacArthur Foundation Research Network on Successful Aging, especially Rowe and Kahn.[13] Rowe and Kahn and their colleagues relied on a largely biological definition of success, denoting good health, high functional capacity, and active engagement. Distressingly, the term came to be used in a normative way, to invoke the vital aging imperative as the standard of success—or failure—for all elders. More recently, Kahn and colleagues acknowledged the unintended normative purposes to which the term has been put and have sought to expand the concept to include social and even subjective measures.[14]

Creative adaptation is also not necessarily vital aging. The latter term was first used by Betty Friedan[15] in a positive sense to counter the "age mystique"; that is, the problematization of aging. The term has also been used in a negative sense, to evoke the contemporary western cultural construct of aging as solely a positive experience, a norm that may be largely inaccessible to immigrant elderly.[16]

Creative adaptation goes beyond both successful aging and vital aging, because it is both an end and a means to an end. We have often met seniors who, in spite of extremely poor health, very impaired functional status, and even lack of social engagement, seem to succeed at aging or to be aging vitally. In cases like these, we see that being successful at aging amounts essentially to coping, adaptation, and resilience (CAR). The CAR construct has best been described by Foster[17] who points out that unlike physical health and function, these mental health functions are well preserved throughout the life span. Foster sketches the implications of the CAR construct for approaches to psychiatric treatment but stops short of promoting CAR as a paradigm for adaptation in aging. It is the work of Wagnild and colleagues that offers the most thorough empirical analysis of the correlation of one component of CAR, namely resilience, showing that it is measurable[18] and that it is correlated with life satisfaction, morale, stress management, lower levels of depression, better health, and health-promoting behaviors.[19]

In keeping with a deliberative model of the professional relationship, the clinician should engage in this active fostering of optimal coping, adaptation, and resilience. How can we do so? By definition, the possibilities are unique and unpredictable. Nonetheless, models for the processes of creative adaptation exist.[20] Such models have similarities, not surprisingly perhaps since human nature is true to itself, with ancient models of self-rediscovery in new and challenging settings. But such articulated models—new and ancient alike—are relatively little used in clinical practice. This gap represents an opportunity for identifying another realistic and ethical imperative. Since quality of existence is the key issue for the elderly and the dying, any significant gap in pursuing it means that there is room for improvement that should be seized as part of the obligation of society to care for elders. Carers should pursue possibilities for creative adaptation for elders. In the realities of elders' lives and carers' approaches, many creative adaptations can be found. An explicit focus on the approach could foster many more.

One model of creative adaptation suggests that after a loss there is an initial stage of cognitive realization. Then, a person tends to withdraw until a deeper understanding and acceptance allows experimentation with different ways to exist in the absence of what has been lost. Only at this point does the person recreate his or her interactions with the world and relationships with people in his or her recreated rendition. For instance, a person may eventually understand and accept that he or she will never again be able to walk or talk or perform activities of daily living, and then may eventually experiment with and discover new ways of negotiating the needs of living and ways of creating meaningful relationships in spite of the disability, either with people from the past or with new people. In the clinical setting, attention to the ways that patients are adapting to adverse circumstances would do much to teach us how to better support the process of adaptation.

For elderly and dying people, the personal and social resources that such creative adaptations demand may be greater than they can manage. But with help and encouragement, people do find ways to adapt to extraordinary circumstances and are often inspiring to those around them as they do so. Thus the clinician who wishes to support the coping, adaptation, and resilience of his or her patients must also pay special attention to the resources—especially social and cultural—that the patients bring to the clinical encounter.

COMPREHENSIVE POPULATION ASSESSMENT:
A BASIS FOR SERVICE PLANNING

If it is apparent that comprehensive individual assessment is the keystone to thorough and therefore effective care, what may be less recognized is that the sum of comprehensive individual assessments constitutes a comprehensive population needs assessment. While many countries and other, smaller jurisdictions have for many years used aggregated needs assessment data to plan service provision, American jurisdictions still lack sufficient information about the numbers of people needing various levels of care to make the tradeoffs among sites of care (between institutional versus community-based care, for example) that are implicit in systematic service planning. We do not mean to imply that no such information is available; in fact, national sample surveys and studies of some important segments of the elderly population (for example, veterans) have gone a good distance to telling us what the structure of an optimal system of care might be. Some have argued that it is impossible to plan for trade-offs between the institutional and non-institutional sectors when there are multiple parallel systems of public and private care and when there are insufficiencies in both sectors. However, in the looming shadow of the baby boom generation, it seems more than ever before incumbent on planners—if only in the public sector—to husband our collective resources by retaining older people in the community for as long as possible.

This is not a new realization, and many states have put one or another assessment mechanism in place. However, until information generated by such assessments can be used to plan services on a community-wide basis, it will have eluded its full potential, and elderly and dying people will land in nursing homes who otherwise—with sufficiently funded community-based services and assisted living settings, for example—would not have to resort to institutional care.

This is particularly true for those people who are highly dependent elderly or dying. Families often go to great lengths and make extraordinary sacrifices—financially, emotionally, and physically—to keep their dependent elderly and dying members at home. The community-based support available to them is often too little (whether measured in hours per day, or by type of care) to support them in providing care, even over the relatively short period of time it is needed. They are forced to seek care through a less expensive gray market, using undocumented aliens as caregivers, or forced to place their elderly family member in a nursing home—a decision that serves neither the needs of the elderly person, the family, nor the needs of society for affordable care. A realistic and ethical approach would be to establish a minimal basis of entitlement to community-based services sufficient to maintain elderly and dying people at home and a minimum amount of such services that will be available, based on comprehensive population assessment. Until this level of services is available, community-based services will be ineffective at keeping people out of nursing homes and thus will be a simulacrum of what they ought to be.

ROLES FOR ELDERS AND THE DYING: A RAISON D'ETRE FOR CREATIVE ADAPTATION IN AGING

Creative adaptation and quality of existence may be assisted by engaging in roles that are reserved specifically for the elderly and for the dying. Roles guide expectations of those engaged in them and of those engaged with the person in the role.[21] Many societies have role-related expectations for elders. These usually include expectations of wisdoms about life that the elder can offer, and expectations of respect that serve to protect the vulnerable elder and to define a relationship in which the "mantle" is passed or legacy given. The loss of elder roles through the devaluation of aging in modern Western society may be contributing to the difficulties elders have in facing the challenges of aging in present times.

The dying also have a role specifically for this life stage, and again, modern Western society may have lost track of this role.[22] The dying role is perhaps an enhanced version of the elders' role in that dying well seems to entail "passing the mantle." It also entails settling differences when possible, saying good-bye, and finishing the last chapter of one's life story as best as is possible. While premature entry to this role can be distressing to the individual and to those who are connected to him or her, and while the role can be misused, the net benefit of having a social understanding of the role so that people can be guided in their expectations (including ethical norms) probably outweighs these risks.

Creative adaptations to aging and dying should be fostered by such role expectations.

For several decades, geriatrics and gerontology have relied on a model which aims to compress morbidity, thus making dying a relatively rapid process.[23] That goal seems to be partly attainable.[24] Because morbidity is undesirable, this is a good thing. But not all of aging is undesirable, and it also seems to be limited by the realities of chronic disease. A revised model based on creative adaptation that seeks quality of existence in role-specific life stages may be a more realistic and more attainable goal for care of the elderly and dying.

The further extension of the three notions advanced above as critical for good care of elders and the dying—goals of care based on a comprehensive assessment and creative adaptation to inevitable real losses—has a public health corollary. A well-discerned approach into the social care of the aging can generate creative solutions in the social setting as well, providing another example of a realistic and ethical approach to the challenges of aging and dying in the current era.

DEMENTIA AND IMPLICATIONS FOR CARE: A TEST CASE FOR REALISTIC AND ETHICAL APPROACHES

This section considers a feature of aging that is paradigmatic and particularly challenging: dementia. Given the stark realities of lost mental capacity, are the imperatives identified above realistic?

Dementia is the single most characteristic and dreaded of aging-related illness. A form of end-organ failure, dementia is among the slowest of the terminal diseases and among the most difficult for the family and community.[25] The suffering of the person with dementia is hard to estimate but surely entails losses in all the areas of personal meaning and often overlaps with physical suffering as well, due to the difficulty in communicating care needs. Often starting with losses in short-term memory and computational speed, people with dementia often transition into disorientation with respect to time and place. Capacity for normal roles in the workplace declines and relationships seem to evaporate. The person with dementia reacts to the losses. During stages of mild to moderate dementia, people describe a sense of diminished respect and complain of being ignored and treated as something less than a person. The losses continue, to include personality changes and, often, maladaptive behaviors including wandering, aggression, and sexual disinhibition. In moderate to late stages of dementia, it becomes difficult to understand the subjective realities of people with dementia, and society tends to stop trying; even carers also stop trying in many cases.

Caregivers struggle to supplement their family member or charge's capacities with their own and often suffer from the diversion from their own life course and from the resulting isolation, exhaustion, and economic losses.[26] Depression and other chronic medical conditions are more common among caregivers of patients with Alzheimer's disease than among matched controls.[27] These caregivers are in many senses the next wave of patients and should be a target for preventive medical strategies.

For those who subscribe to the compression of morbidity hypothesis as an approach to aging well and dying well, dementia is the ultimate challenge. While dementia is mild, creative adaptations to minimize morbidity are possible through creative living arrangements, but the overall picture is one of a slow, inexorable slide toward severe dementia. Newer anticholinergic and other agents that seem to slow the decline only stave off the inevitable. After the early stages, this smooth trajectory has no plateau at which morbidity can be compressed, nor any in which it transitions promptly to mortality. Moderate dementia arrives with its greater challenges to personhood and greater physical suffering as well as greater challenges to the caregivers.

A few approaches to the care of persons with dementia seem to have realistic and ethical merit. One approach is essentially palliative care in the long-term care setting of choice (i.e., at home or in institutions); that is, judicious use of medical interventions with advance care planning discussions, to come as close as possible to a natural and comfortable dignified dying. Reliance on advance care planning with dementia patients is not always possible, especially when they come to the care facility already advanced in dementia. However, family members can sometimes be of assistance here, and most want nothing more than dignified palliative care. Other approaches to the care of persons with dementia have been explored in geriatrics. They focus on the creation of relational meaning between carers and patients by meeting the patient where the condition has taken him or her.[28] Such approaches have implications for every aspect of care, from medical and nursing care to the planning of activities and meals, to dealing with problematic behaviors. The rise of special dementia care units in nursing homes across the country has been especially helpful in bringing together people with the disease, their families, and professionals who wish to devote their energies to the improvement of care of this population.

Judicious Use of Life-Prolonging Interventions

Life-sustaining interventions can be withheld for persons with dementia, while full palliative care can ensure some comfort and dignity, to capture the natural exits that normal life provides. But conventional care allows many moderately demented people to live well enough that no natural exits arrive or if they do, are seemingly easily overcome with antibiotics or other readily available interventions. People with dementia thus live on to reach the stages of severe dementia, bypassing the compressed morbidity option entirely. The natural instincts of human beings to avoid death both for ourselves and those for whom we care makes this seem an immediate ethical imperative, and yet with a broader view, perhaps a missed ethical option.

The advance care planning option has been proposed as an answer to this ethical quagmire, only to be countered with the problems of changing personhood status and changing wishes so that the authenticity of advanced wishes is unclear.[29] Ideally, we should obtain advance directives much in advance of the onset of dementia. We must also deal more explicitly with the designation of responsibility for health care decision making, for when the designation is unclear, decisions often cannot be reached. No better option has yet revealed itself than to rely dually on the affected persons' earlier-expressed wishes and on the current wishes of an expressly designated proxy decision-maker.

Palliative Care in the Long-Term Care Setting

The ethical claims made on the society to care for those of our members who have dementia may be balanced against the rest of the population's needs, but the claims are nevertheless legitimate and will not go away. Those of us who have dementia have a strong claim to care that treats us with dignity and that finds creative ways to adapt the caring options available to us as well as the settings in which we can live to our special needs. The obligation continues until such time that the patient (or the proxy if authority has been transferred) either faces inevitable death or death from an illness for which life-sustaining intervention can be ethically withheld. The ethical imperative for elders with dementia is therefore still the same as it always has been, although embellished with new options brought by information technology and other advanced devices, namely to provide types of long-term care, whether in the home, in the community, or in institutions, which provide a dignified quality of life for the elders affected and that can be sustained by the population.[30]

At the present time, much of palliative care has focused on populations suffering from conditions other than dementia. The current ethical imperative is therefore to explore how locations where the persons with dementia live—home or long-term care—can access palliative care, and how palliative care can to be adapted to address the needs of these groups.[31] Nearly every hospice has service agreements with multiple nursing homes, and most nursing homes are now contracted with one or more hospices.[32] Yet, the synergistic potential between the two organizations—hospice and nursing homes—has yet to be explored, and indeed, conflicts can arise between the two forms of care. Most importantly, collaborations between the two types of organizations would do well to focus on identifying the appropriate point of onset of palliative care for chronic illnesses, since studies show that the typical length of stay in hospice is so short as to obviate any potential benefit.

Creating Relational Meaning in Caregiving

In the context of long-term care, one of the creative adaptation approaches that adds optimism to a particularly glum vista is that which focuses on creating a meeting place of meaning between the patient and the carer. In a brightly illustrative example of this, the American Psychiatric Nurses Association[33] has documented the revolution in the lives of an elderly woman with dementia and her carer around bath time. In the pre-intervention phase, bath time was a troublesome matter to both parties, a time in which the patient often became combative. In the intervention, the carers brainstormed about and were able to glean insight into the perspective of the patient, whom they understood to need more dignity and control and for whom they found ways to offer it. After experimenting with different options, the result was a moving scene in which bath time became a time when affection was exchanged between the two women, one demented and dependent, the other capable and caring. For this interaction both received the meaning and dignity that accompany exchanged gifts of human affection.

The key to providing humanistic long-term care for those with dementia may well be that meaning is relational and relational meaning is likely possible for many people with dementia, so long as the time and effort necessary to understand their perspective is taken. As with so many other interventions, the time and effort expended is significant but probably an excellent investment in terms of subsequent quality of life for the patient and in fulfillment for the caregiving professional and hence retention of employees by service delivery organizations. While it is unusual to cast meaning creation in ethical terms, to the extent that meaning creation is part of engaging in relationships that offer the dignity of personhood, this may indeed be the core of the ethical imperative for elders with dementia.

THE SOCIAL SETTING OF AGING: ARE REALISTIC AND ETHICAL RESPONSES POSSIBLE?

This section examines some of the dilemmas that are posed by the sociodemographic bulge caused by the large birth rate immediately after World War II and that now has yielded a well-cared for and therefore increasingly old population.

Seventy-seven million baby boomers are planning for their soon-to-arrive retirement. For the first time in this country's history, the United States has more elderly than children in its population. If current trends continue, the 65-and-over population will have tripled by the end of the decade, while the under-65 population will have shrunk to one-third of what it was at the start of the decade. This ballooning of the elderly population requires unprecedented planning for the inevitable medical, economic, and social consequences.

Most individuals are, at best, prepared for economic life in retirement according to old models in which Social Security and Medicare would be adequate safety nets. This is no longer realistic. Further, the private sector's ability to absorb part of the health care costs of retirees is questionable. Almost half of the country's large employers have imposed financial caps on their retiree benefit obligations, something that was almost unheard of in the 1990s.

The "sandwich generation" that currently faces the cost of educating children and caring for dependent elders will give way to a new version of the same, in which the dependent elders will be more numerous and older than ever, with some middle-aged individuals caring for grandparents and great grandparents. The ratio of working Americans to retired Americans is currently about five workers for every one retiree. By current trends, in the 2030s the ratio will be two or three workers per retiree.[34]

Similarly, decades of study on aging at the cellular and molecular level may now be coming together with clinical and social research and policy to achieve some progress toward the "holy grail" of extended longevity. For longer life to be something better than an exacerbation of the demographic catastrophe threatened by aging baby boomers, enhanced models for elders and seriously ill people that entail creative adaptation and economic productivity until the last possible moment are likely necessary.[35]

Society-wide Creative Adaptations

Given the ethical imperative described above and the uniquely challenging medical needs of elders, creative adaptations on the part of society as well as on the part of individuals and carers are essential.

The outlook most likely to generate creative adaptations that are viable is that which sees the problem as an opportunity. Elders are older and healthier than ever before. To quote the wisdom of one visionary, William Beveridge, who led the effort to create the National Health Service in Britain: "There is no reason . . . to doubt the power of large numbers of people to go on working with advantage to the community and happiness to themselves after reaching the minimum pensionable age. . . . The natural presumption for the increasing length of total life is that the length of years during which working capacity lasts will also rise. . . . A people ageing in years need not be old in spirit."[36] In similar spirit, Ken Dychtwald noted: "We haven't yet figured out the modern purpose of a healthier old age. To what use do we put the incredible resource of elderhood?"[37]

The ethical imperative is an imaginative tool. What is also needed is innovation that can point the way from delineating the problem to proposing a solution. A proposed solution would recognize that what we face is, in essence, a lengthening time span of human productivity. If we can properly restructure workplace duties and rewards (particularly salary and benefits), we can create a situation where the working elderly, employers, and society as a whole will gain from the continued relationship. Key considerations include:

- Elders are more functional and in better health than ever before.
- More elders want to work.
- The range of possible roles for elders should reflect their accumulated experience and wisdom on the one hand and their declining energy and abilities on the other.
- Salaries and personal expenditures should decline after a peak in earlier years, rather than climb until retirement.

Palliative Care as a Social Intervention

One approach that may have more creativity in it than has yet been tapped is that of palliative care. Palliative care is founded on the notion that the whole person suffers, so the whole person, in their context of family and community, is the unit of care. Palliative care attends to the psychological, social, existential, and physical aspects of life of the patient and family and community. It relies on low technology interventions that draw on an interdisciplinary team.[38] The impact of palliative care on quality of life has been impressive enough that it has become a veritable movement in medicine. But the aspect of palliative care that may remain unappreciated has to do with its economics. The cost of care near the end of life has received considerable attention, in part because health care expenditures near the end of life exceed those incurred in the rest of life put together.[39] But what seems to have gone largely unnoticed is that scholarly analyses of medical costs are focused exclusively on direct costs and omit the area that is most characteristic of the palliative care approach: indirect costs. The impact of palliative care on keeping a patient active until the last possible moment, keeping the caregiver supported and active throughout their caregiving role, and preparing and supporting them during bereavement so that they recover well and remain active members of society are all lost to the existing economic analyses.[40] It is entirely possible that the palliative care paradigm will be most suited to solving the puzzle of how to care for the elderly in the most cost-effective way by also attending to their social and economic needs.

Economic Development By, For, and In Services to the Elderly

There is another reality buried in this approach, namely that the type of care needed by elderly and dying people could promote the development of a service provider industry that relies on relatively low-skilled labor, namely caregivers and the ability of the system to produce its own new labor force automatically in that family members of patients have to learn caregiving skills for their own family members. A caregiving certification program that builds on that in-home learning could yield a devoted labor force that can tailor its capacity to its own physical limitations by working within its local community.

A variation on the theme breaks away from the palliative care paradigm and yet uses the notion that elders are capable of a wide range of contributions to society, illness and disability notwithstanding. So long as mental capacity is intact, use of information technology and other devices to assist with declining physical capacity should be able to yield a productive elder workforce. What is needed is a set of programs that foster elders' own creativity. In one sense, the growing threat to the survival of Social Security, the Medicare crisis, and the growing difficulty of putting aside savings for retirement years are all driving creative adaptation as elders seek ways to provide for their last years.

So, as the imperative to care and the rising tide of need come face to face, there is an opportunity to seize. Society could hide its face in the characteristically modern flight from aging and from the aged. Or, we could embrace the ethical charge to venerate our elders and, embracing not only their wisdom but also their capacity for contribution, we could ride this sociodemographic wave into new enlightenment. It is the only approach that is both realistic and ethical.

NOTES

1. James R. Knickman and Emily K. Snell, "2030 Problem: Caring for Aging Baby Boomers," *Health Services Research* 37 (2002): 849–84. See also D. P. Rice and N. Fineman, "Economic Implications of Increased Longevity in the United States," *Annual Review of Public Health* 25 (2004): 457–73; and M. Evandrou, *Baby Boomers: Ageing in the 21st Century* (London: Age Concern England, 1997). See also Elizabeth Benedict, "When Baby Boomers Grow Old," *American Prospect* 12, no. 9 (2001): 1–20.

2. Liz Lloyd, "Mortality and Morality: Ageing and the Ethics of Care," *Aging & Society* 24 (2004): 235–56.

3. Robert Kastenbaum, *Psychology of Death*, 3rd ed. (New York: Springer, 2000). C. Rocke and K. E. Cherry, "Death at the End of the 20th Century: Individual Processes and Developmental Tasks in Old Age." *International Journal of Aging and Human Development* 54, no. 4 (2002): 315–33.

4. C. E. Sluzki, "Social Networks and the Elderly: Conceptual and Clinical Issues, and a Family Consultation," *Family Process* 39, no. 3 (2000): 271–84.

5. V. G. Cicirelli, "Older Adults' Fear and Acceptance of Death: A Transition Model," *Ageing International* 28, no. 1 (2003): 66–81.

6. F. T. Sherman, "'I Want to Die': Pseudo-Death Wishes and the Search for Joy in the Older Population," *Geriatrics* 57, no. 10 (2002): 8–9.

7. M. Nakashima and E. R. Canda, "Positive Dying and Resiliency in Later Life: A Qualitative Study," *Journal of Aging Studies* 19 (2005): 109–25.

8. M. Gillick, S. Berkman, and L. Cullen, "Patient-Centered Approach to Advance Medical Planning in the Nursing Home," *Journal of the American Geriatrics Society* 47, no. 2 (1999): 227–30. See also W. E. Haley, R. S. Allen, S. Reynolds, H. Chen, A. Burton, and D. Gallagher-Thompson, "Family Issues in End-of-Life Decision-Making and End-of-Life Care." *American Behavioral Scientist* 46, no. 2 (2002): 284–98.

9. E. J. Emanuel and L. L. Emanuel, "Four Models of the Doctor-Patient Relationship," *Journal of the American Medical Association* 267 (1992): 2067–71. See also G. S. Fisher, H. R. Alpert, J. D. Stoeckle, and L. L. Emanuel, "Can Goals of Care Be Used to Predict Intervention Preferences in an Advance Directive?" *Archives of Internal Medicine* 157 (1997): 801–7.

10. L. L. Emanuel, "The Hippocratic Oath," *Journal of Clinical Ethics* 1, no. 4 (1991): 273–74.

11. C. Santina Della and R. H. Bernstein, "Whole-Patient Assessment, Goal Planning, and Inflection Points: Their Role in Achieving Quality End-of-Life Care," *Clinics in Geriatric Medicine* 20 (2004): 595–620.

12. M. A. Camann and L. Chase, "Older Adults: The Case for Comprehensive Assessment," *Caring* 20, no. 1 (2001): 26–28.

13. J. W. Rowe and R. L. Kahn, *Successful Aging: The MacArthur Foundation Study* (New York: Pantheon, 1998).

14. L. W. Poon, S. H. Gueldner, and B. M. Sprouse, *Successful Aging and Adaptation with Chronic Diseases* (New York: Springer, 2003).

15. B. Friedan, *Fountain of Age* (New York: Simon & Schuster, 1993).

16. C. Berdes and A. A. Zych, "Subjective Quality of Life of Polish, Polish-Immigrant, and Polish-American Elderly," *International Journal of Aging and Human Development* 50, no. 4 (2000): 385–95.

17. J. R. Foster, "Successful Coping, Adaptation and Resilience in the Elderly: An Interpretation of Epidemiologic Data," *Psychiatric Quarterly* 68, no. 3 (1997): 189–219.

18. G. M. Wagnild and H. M. Young, "Development and Psychometric Evaluation of the Resilience Scale," *Journal of Nursing Management* 1, no. 2 (1993): 165–78.

19. Wagnild and Young, "Development and Psychometric Evaluation of the Resilience Scale." See also G. M. Wagnild, "Resilience and Successful Aging: Comparison among Low and High-Income Older Adults," *Journal of Gerontological Nursing* 29, no. 12 (2003): 42–49.

20. H. Q. Kivnick and S. V. Murray, "Life Strengths Interview Guide: Assessing Elder Clients' Strengths," *Journal of Gerontological Social Work* 34, no. 4 (2001): 7–32.

21. D. L. Infeld, *Sociology of Aging,* vol. 3, *Disciplinary Approaches to Aging* (New York: Routledge, 2002).

22. H. G. Prigerson, "Socialization to Dying: Social Determinants of Death Acknowledgment and Treatment among Terminally Ill Geriatric Patients," *Journal of Health and Social Behavior* 33, no. 4 (1992): 378–95.

23. J. M. Laditka and S. B. Laditka, "Morbidity Compression Debate: Risks, Opportunities, and Policy Options for Women," *Journal of Women and Aging* 12, nos. 1–2 (2000): 23–38.

24. M. L. Daviglus, K. Liu, A. Pirzada, et al., "Favorable Cardiovascular Risk Profile in Middle Age and Health-Related Quality of Life in Older Age," *Archives of Internal Medicine* 163 (2003): 2460–68.

25. C. von Gunten and D. E. Weissman, "Information for Patients and Families about Ventilator Withdrawal," *Journal of Palliative Medicine* 6, no. 5 (2003): 775–76.

26. I. I. Kneebone and P. R. Martin, "Coping and Caregivers of People with Dementia," *British Journal of Health Psychology* 8, no. 1 (2003): 1–17. See also H. Brodaty, A. Green, and A. Koschera, "Meta-Analysis of Psychosocial Interventions for Caregivers of People with Dementia," *Journal of the American Geriatrics Society* 51, no. 5 (2003): 657–64.

27. D. V. Powers, D. Gallagher-Thompson, and H. C. Kraemer, "Coping and Depression in Alzheimer's Caregivers: Longitudinal Evidence of Stability," *Journals of Gerontology: Series B: Psychological Sciences and Social Sciences* 57B, no. 3 (2002): P205–11. See also P. C. Clark and K. B. King, "Comparison of Family Caregivers: Stroke Survivors vs. Persons with Alzheimer's Disease," *Journal of*

Gerontological Nursing 29, no. 2 (2003): 45–53; and J. R. Shua-Haim, T. Haim, Y. Shi, Y-H Kuo, and J. M. Smith, "Depression among Alzheimer's Caregivers: Identifying Risk Factors," *American Journal of Alzheimer's Disease and Other Dementias* 16, no. 6 (2001): 353–59.

28. J. M. Zgola, *Care That Works: A Relationship Approach to Persons with Dementia* (Baltimore, Md.: Johns Hopkins University Press, 1999).

29. J. Vollman, "Advance Directives in Patients with Alzheimer's Disease: Ethical and Clinical Considerations," *Medicine, Health Care, Philosophy* 4, no. 2 (2001): 161–67.

30. S. G. Post, "Fear of Forgetfulness: A Grassroots Approach to an Ethics of Alzheimer's Disease," *Journal of Clinical Ethics* 9, no. 1 (1998): 71–80.

31. S. C. Miller, J. Teno, and V. Mor, "Hospice and Palliative Care in Nursing Homes," *Clinics in Geriatric Medicine* 20 (2004): 717–34.

32. K. N. Rice, E. A. Coleman, R. Fish, C. Levy, and J. S. Kutner, "Factors Influencing Models of End-of-Life Care in Nursing Homes: Results of a Survey of Nursing Home Administrators," *Journal of Palliative Medicine* 4, no. 5 (2004): 668–75.

33. American Psychiatric Nurses Association, "Choice and Challenge: Caring for Aggressive Older Adults Across Levels of Care," (film). Coproduced by Terra Nova Films and Abbe, Inc. (1998) and available at http://www.terranova.org.

34. Social Security Administration. *The 2004 OASDI Trustees Report of the Board of Trustees of the Federal Old-Age and Survivors Insurance and Disability.*

35. B. A. Butrica, R. W. Johnson, K. E. Smith, and E. Steuerle, *Does Work Pay at Older Ages?* (Washington, D.C.: The Urban Institute, 2004).

36. W. Beveridge, *Social Insurance and Allied Services*, the Beveridge Report (London: HMSO, 1942).

37. K. Dychtwald, "The Ten Physical, Social, Spiritual, Economic, and Political Crises the Boomers Will Face as They Age in the 21st Century," http://www.as aging.org/am/cia/dychtwald.html (March 29, 2005).

38. L. L. Emanuel, C. Alexander, R. M. Arnold, et al., (Palliative Care Guidelines Group of the American Hospice Foundation), "Integrating Palliative Care into Disease Management Guidelines," *Journal of Palliative Medicine* 7, no. 6 (2004): 774–83.

39. J. Lubitz, L. Cai, E. Kramarow, and H. Lentzner, "Health, Life Expectancy, and Health Care Spending among the Elderly," *New England Journal of Medicine* 349 (2003): 1048–55.

40. A. A. Boni–Saenz, D. Dranove, L. L. Emanuel, and A. T. Lo Sasso, "The Price of Palliative Care: Toward a Complete Accounting of Costs and Benefits," *Clinics in Geriatric Medicine* 21 (2005): 147–63.

Rage, Rage against the Dying of the Light: Not a Metaphor for End-of-Life Care

John J. Paris, Michael D. Schreiber, and Robert Fogerty

Do not go gentle into that good night.
Old age should burn and rage at the close of day.
Rage, rage against the dying of the light.

Though wise men at their end know dark is right,
Because their words had forked no lightning they
Do not go gentle into the good night.

Good men, the last wave by, crying how bright
Their frail deeds might have danced in a green bay,
Rage, rage against the dying of the light.

Wild men who caught and sang the sun in flight,
And learn, too late, they grieved it on its way,
Do not go gentle into that good night.

Grave men, near death, who see with blinding sight,
Blind eyes could blaze like meteors and be gay,
Rage, rage against the dying of the light.

And you, my father, there on the sad height,
Curse, bless me now with your fierce tears, I pray.
Do not go gentle into that good night.
Rage, rage against the dying of the light.[1]

These words of Dylan Thomas exhorting his dying father not to give up but to fight and rage against death are gripping poetry. Oft quoted, they signal a determination that over and against the sure knowledge of inevitable death the good, the strong, yes even the wise thing to do is to struggle. Struggle not in the hope of defeating death, but in the firm resolve to die as one lived, fighting fiercely. Of such action is greatness defined, heroes formed.

The difficulty with the metaphor and the impulse to make it normative at the end-of-life is that, other than in military action, heroic battle against death is rarely marked with anything but pain and prolonged suffering. Indeed, at the twilight of a long life or the end stage of a terminal disease even Dylan Thomas concedes that "wise men know dark is right." Death in those situations is not an enemy. It is simply a part of the human condition, a mark of what it means to be mortal. The modern unwillingness to accept that reality leads to the illusion noted by Daniel Callahan that if only we push hard enough medicine will triumph not only over disease, but over death itself.[2]

Immortality, however, was not Dylan Thomas's goal. He readily acknowledges that the fading light ultimately dissolves into darkness, whatever that darkness signifies. The challenge today is how to distinguish the struggle against the forces of human diminishment—old age, sickness and disease—from a continuing struggle when, having exerted all our energy and resources, the body will still succumb to death. How, we must ask ourselves, do we recognize and respond to the dying process?

The all too frequent demand in today's end-of life care to "do everything possible" is an understandable plea not to give up on a patient when medical intervention offers a small but real possibility of reversing the disease process. The ethical issue, however, is what to do when the prognosis shifts from "possible" to "dim" to "dismal." In the face of those changed circumstances, is the physician still obliged to respond positively to the request to use every technological means available to prolong the patient's life?

HISTORICAL BACKGROUND

Within the Western Hippocratic tradition the answer is clearly "no." The treatise entitled *The Art* in the Hippocratic Corpus defines medicine as having three roles: "Doing away with the suffering of the sick, lessening the violence of their diseases, and refusing to treat those overmastered by their diseases, realizing that in such cases medicine is powerless."[3] In pointed terms, Hippocrates goes even further when he declares, "To impose treatment on the patient overmastered by disease is to display an ignorance akin to madness."[4]

The tradition of limiting the use of medical interventions in the face of impending death was broadened and strengthened through some four hundred years of moral reflection on the duty to preserve life. Beginning with the teaching of Domingo Soto in the sixteenth century that religious superiors could only require their subjects to use medicine that could be taken without too much difficulty through the Vatican's *1980 Declaration of Euthanasia*[5] and Pope John Paul II's encyclical *Evangelican Vitae,*[6] there has been a continuing emphasis on the right of the patient to decline what in the older terminology was called "extraordinary" means.[7] That term, as the President's Commission's Report on *Deciding to Forego Life Sustaining Technology* notes, has become so misused and abused that it is no longer useful in public policy discourse.[8] In its place, the President's Commission proposed adopting the Vatican *Declaration's* emphasis on "proportionate and disproportionate burden and benefit" analysis.

Here both the President's Commission and the Vatican are reverting to the traditional distinction between "ordinary" and "extraordinary" first proposed in 1595 by Domingo Banez. The theological understanding of the terms refers not to technique, hardware, or ease of administration, but to the duty every individual has to preserve his or her life. In the theological context in which these terms were developed, the duty was a moral one. Failure to observe that duty in an important matter would be a mortal sin, the punishment for which, if not absolved before death, was consignment to hell. With the threat of eternal damnation at stake, the immediate question became, "what excused one from the obligation to undertake medical treatment?" The answer provided by the moral theologians was clear: There was no duty to undergo any treatment that was too costly, too painful, too burdensome or any treatment no matter how simple, readily available, or inexpensive that did not offer an expectation of significant benefit to the patient.

Paul Ramsey's 1970 essay "On (Only) Caring for the Dying," adopted and updated those standards.[9] In his essay, Ramsey acknowledged the fact that the moral and the medical communities had different understandings of the terms "ordinary" and "extraordinary." For physicians, the term "extraordinary" took on the connotation of something difficult, rare, or exceedingly expensive. Such procedures might legitimately be rejected by the patient. But in the mind of the medical community, the physician's commitment to the patient's well-being meant that the physician also had a duty to use things that were simple, readily available, and easy to administer, such as antibiotics and intravenous feeding.

Historically, however, the words "extraordinary" and "ordinary" referred to the patient's duties, not the physician's. Nor did the terms ever refer to technique or ease of use. The basis of the obligation, rather, was the proportionate benefit-burden experienced by the patient from the use of intervention. If in the patient's subjective assessment the benefit was not worth the pain and suffering, there was no moral duty to institute or continue the treatment.

In the circumstances of an imminently dying patient, Ramsey proposed that aggressive medical interventions were not only not obligatory, their imposition was an abuse. The proper treatment for the dying patient should not be to offer "pretended remedies," but to offer comfort and company. Holding the patient's hand and being present to company with him or her on the final stages of life's journey are the most that can be done for the dying patient, and so for Ramsey, as was true of the Hippocratic physician, care at the end of life is to provide the patient with comfort and company.

Ramsey's essay was patient oriented. The expectation of his pastoral approach was that neither the patient nor the physician, once they understood the dying process had been entered into, would insist on continuing aggressive medical treatments. The "technological imperative," the notion that if we have a technology available it must be used—indifferent to efficiency or cost—had yet to take hold. Not until the 1970s was there the technical means, or even the thought, that maintaining an individual in the dying process—or an irreversible comatose state—was a desirable goal.

Writing on the topic of end-of-life care in the 1950s, Gerald Kelly, the foremost moral theologian of his era, noted that he was frequently asked by physicians whether one must provide oxygen and intravenous feedings to a patient in what he described as a "terminal coma."[10] Kelly's response is instructive: "Once the condition is well diagnosed, not only is there no obligation to provide them, to do so is wrong: there is no benefit to patient, there is great tension on family, and expense to community."[11] Note that it is the physician who is called upon to make a decision on discontinuing a technique that could but prolong a comatose existence. In Kelly's judgment there is no question of the moral character of continuing a medical means to extend the life of a patient in an unending comatose state: it is wrong.

Richard McCormick, another Jesuit moralist, in a landmark article published in JAMA (1974) entitled "To Live or Let Die" gives a theological explanation for the legitimacy of withholding or withdrawing life-prolonging treatments from patients who are so compromised that they face either imminent death or a life suffused in suffering.[12] As he explains, the Christian tradition understands life as a gift from God whose purpose is relationship with God and fellow humans. If the potential for those relationships is precluded by the absence of consciousness or so hampered by endless struggles merely to survive that it cannot flourish, then the purpose of that life—no matter how extended or brief its duration—has been fulfilled. When that point is reached there is no further warrant for prolonging the life; its earthly goal has been achieved.

THE MODERN ERA

Modern medical technology, which can postpone death indefinitely, poses a challenge to the approach that prevailed in Western culture from the time of Hippocrates up through the middle of the twentieth century. That reality is captured in Edmund Pellegrino's division of medicine into three eras: Hippocrates to 1960; 1960–1990; 1990 to the present.[13] The view that "nature" set a limit on what could or should be done to preserve life prevailed until about 1960. Prior to that time, all that medicine could provide was found in the doctor's little black bag: a stethoscope, a tongue depressor, a rubber mallet to test neurologic response, and a few antibiotics. Beyond observing, listening, diagnosing, and comforting, there was precious little a doctor could do in the face of a life-threatening condition.

The era from 1960–1990 changed all that. Technological advances from ventilators and organ transplantation to genetic manipulation allowed doctors to push back the barriers to extending life. "Miracle cures" were discovered, diseases eradicated, and once "hopeless" cases came to be seen as merely challenges. These advances, coupled with universal third party coverage for those hospitalized with an acute illness, gave rise to new expectations and new demands among patients. Nothing, it seemed, was beyond our grasp. Disease could be destroyed and death defeated if only we worked hard enough to discover the means of doing so.

Along with the development of technology and third party payment to cover its costs, another factor loomed large in the period from 1960–1990: the breakdown of institutional authority. Physician paternalism and patient submission to "the doctor knows best" philosophy gave way to a consumer oriented approach to medicine. The physician's role now was to provide whatever the patient (or surrogate) demanded.

As Pellegrino laments, the result in this shift of thinking has been chaos. Unregulated and unrestrained medical consumerism sustained the belief that so long as the medical service is paid for the doctor should do whatever is requested. The 1991 federal Patient Self-Determination Act, which was designed to assure that health care institutions inform patients of their rights under the various state standards to decline unwarranted medical treatments, came to mean in the mind of patients and families that the individual alone determines the intensity and duration of aggressive intervention to prolong life.

Once medicine achieved the ability to prolong life well beyond what "nature" would have deemed proper, many began to reevaluate the proper limits of medicine. The questions that physicians and patients began to address were: Does the extension of a life suffused in suffering make sense? Ought we prolong a life that will never be conscious or never experience human relationships? What is the quality of life we are saving? When is it appropriate to let the patient being overwhelmed by disease die?

There is no question today that if a dying patient rejects aggressive life-sustaining medical treatments, such measures will be withheld or withdrawn. The competent patient's right to do so was acknowledged in the United States Supreme Court's 1990 *Cruzan* opinion where Chief Justice William Rehnquist writing for the Court stated, "The principle that a competent person has a constitutionally protected liberty interest in refusing unwanted medical treatment may be inferred from our prior decisions."[14] The *Cruzan* court also acknowledged that—depending on the evidentiary standards enacted by the various states—proxy judgments to limit or refuse any and all unwanted medical interventions may be made for incompetent patients. But the court left unresolved the more subtle and complex issue of how physicians should respond to patient or family requests for treatments that physicians believed to be medically ineffective or inappropriate.

Initially, the scope of this latter issue seemed rather limited. It focused on simple questions, such as whether a physician should comply with patient requests for antibiotics for viral infections or CT scans for routine headaches. Although theoretically agreeing that such treatments ought not to be provided, many physicians found it easier to go along with patient requests than to try to persuade them otherwise. The "placebo effect" would frequently convince patients they felt better and the insurance company would pay for the treatment. That approach, though, fed the "consumer" mind-set toward medicine on the part of both the patient and the physician. It also contributed to the erosion of physician authority and, more importantly, of professional responsibility.

Still, so long as requests for medical interventions involved rather innocuous medications such as B-12 shots or relatively simple and inexpensive technologies, there was no concern on the part of medicine. But as the "consumer" model began to dominate, the requests escalated into demands for more and more exotic and inappropriate treatments. The belief began to grow that informed consent and patient autonomy implied that patients not only had the right to accept or reject proposed therapies, they had the "right" to propose the therapy itself.

Autonomy, or the right of self-determination, was seen not only as a significant moral principle, but became, in the minds of some bioethicists[15] the overriding moral principle. Other values such as the physician's concern for the well-being of the patient, or the physician's responsibility to "do no harm" became subsidiary to the patient's personal assessment of "benefits and burdens." Even issues of social justice were subordinated to the idiosyncratic demands of the individual patient.

THE CLINICAL QUANDARY

The emphasis on consumerism and informed consent encouraged the belief that respect for autonomy requires the physician to do whatever the patient or family desires. And this, in turn, left many physicians facing a clinical quandary: Is there any limit to the physician's obligation to honor a patient's demands for treatment? Must the physician, if asked, always employ all available means to preserve life? Some physicians find it difficult to place limits on their patients' requests for medical interventions. For example, Dr. Joel Frader of the University of Pittsburgh reports that he feels like "tearing my hair out when a family insists on treatment I think is nuts."[16] Then he asks, "But who am I to think it's nuts? Why should I have more authority than family members of patients?" And still other physicians worry about the ways in which medical consumerism works to undermine sound clinical judgment. Consider the scenario described by Dr. Stanley Friel, in which a young patient dying of cystic fibrosis was accepted "for evaluation" by a transplant center even though he had already passed the threshold of viability as a candidate for a heart-lung transplant.[17] Dr. Friel reported that this action was taken not in the hope of doing the transplant, but so the family would be assured they had done "everything possible." The patient, after a long and stressful cross-country flight, arrived at the hospital in respiratory failure. He died soon thereafter far from home and familiar surroundings.

THE FUTILITY DEBATE

Does the physician's respect for the patient's right of self-determination require the abandonment of clinical judgment in order to honor the patient or the family's desires? This question has been at the core of what has come to be called "the futility debate" in medicine. While we joined in the "futility debate," we have now come to believe that the debate is fatuous, a modern day relapse into nominalism. Though the medical literature is replete with articles titled "Medical Futility: Its Meaning and Ethical Implications";[18] "The Problem with Futility";[19] "Who Defines Futility?";[20] "The Illusion of Futility in Clinical Practice";[21] "Beyond Futility";[22] and "Beyond Futility to an Ethics of Care,"[23] there is no agreement on what the term means or what implications it conveys. Does it signify absolute impossibility?[24] Is it purely physiological? Does it include the ability to revive heartbeat but not to achieve discharge from the hospital? How much quality of life and social value does the term embrace?

One reason for this confusion is that physicians often disagree on both the chances of success and on the goals of therapy. Some invoke futility only if the success rate is zero percent, whereas others declare a treatment futile with a success rate as high as 18 percent. Further, social and psychological factors may cloud a physician's estimate of success. For example, some consider liver transplantation for an alcoholic patient futile because of the likelihood of recidivism. Others believe a treatment futile if all it can provide is a chance for a couple of days or weeks in an intensive care unit.

In 1990, Schneiderman et al. attempted to resolve the confusion over the meaning of futility by proposing a quantitative definition for the term. For them futility refers to "any effort to achieve a result that is possible, but that reasoning or experience suggests is highly improbable and cannot be systematically produced."[25] Schneiderman and colleagues proposed as a rule of thumb, that a treatment should be considered futile if it can be shown not to have worked in the last one hundred cases. The same should be true if the treatment fails to restore consciousness or alleviate total dependence on intensive care. That approach, though a handy rule, is open to serious criticism, however. First, in relation to whose goals is the treatment useless—the patient's or the physician's?[26] Second, what physicians have the practical experience with one hundred cases of a similar nature that would enable them to make such an assessment? And finally, the definition of quantitative futility ignores the fact that, as in the *Wanglie* case, some families might elect treatment that preserves permanent unconsciousness or total dependence on ICU care, particularly when the alternative is death.[27]

In the clinical setting, this lack of agreement on the meaning of futility provides a "shorthand" way for physicians to truncate discussions on treatment decisions. This is one of the real problems with relying on the term. Indeed, jettisoning this new buzzword would be no loss. The debate on "futility" not only distracts, but it also distorts the real issue.

For, it is not the meaning of a word, but the moral basis of the participant's actions that ought to be the focus of our attention.

REFRAMING THE DEBATE

There are two fundamental issues to be faced by physicians, hospitals, and families in cases where a physician believes a requested treatment is unwarranted. These are (1) what is the appropriate medical care for the patient and (2) what is the appropriate response to a patient or a family member who insists on struggling against all odds and all medical evidence to block impending death.

Medical decision making at the end of life is neither an issue of physician domination nor of complete patient self-determination. These determinations are not exclusively scientific judgments; they are, rather, value assumptions about the nature and value of mortal life. As such, they belong to a broader community than medicine alone. The question is not *whether* but *which* value judgments physicians may use in determining whether to follow patient demands. And that question signals a turn away from individual toward social conceptions of the reasonableness and worthwhileness of the proposed procedure.[28] It is neither the personal predilections of the provider nor the idiosyncratic views of the patient, but the common social senses of the approved practices that should prevail. Without this social consensus on the values and ends that undergird medical practice, we will inevitably and unfortunately be forced to turn increasingly to judicial and governmental involvement in these decisions.

To achieve social support for the acceptance of medical standards, physicians' professional societies should provide well-reasoned substantive guidelines for their practice policies. One example can be found in the criteria for the treatment of profoundly compromised or neurologically devastated patients that have already been developed by the President's Commission and by multiple specialty societies.[29] These medical groups agree with the President's Commission that the only justification for instituting or continuing aggressive medical interventions on such patients is the judgment by the physician that the treatment will be effective in restoring the patient to consciousness. Without that expectation not only is there no obligation to proceed with aggressive medical treatments, but the physician has no mandate from either society or the profession to do so.

There are, of course, risks in granting physicians the authority to set medical standards that will prevail against patient or family requests for life-sustaining interventions. And the potential for abuse demands safeguards to ensure that appeal to prevailing standards alone is not a sufficient basis to override treatment requests. Minimally, such decisions should be openly made, principled, and focused on the patient. They should also include agreement among the health care providers, the concurrence of an ethics committee, openness to a second opinion, willingness to cooperate in the transfer of the patient, and sound documentation in a permanent medical record.

A PROCEDURAL APPROACH TO FUTILITY

These procedural safeguards are the mechanism several professional medical groups and two state legislatures have adopted as a response to family-physician disputes over the continuance of aggressive therapies in end-stage or neurologically devastated patients. These associations recognize "that there is no consensus in our society on the meaning of the term futility and that in the absence of such consensus, the problem of making decisions about treatments offering minimal benefit has not disappeared."[30]

Technologic advances over the last two decades have given patients and families the "illusion of control" over life and death.[31] The advances sometimes prove to be but a "halfway" technology—they can stave off death but cannot restore the patient to what the *Dinnerstein* court describes as "cognitive functioning existence."[32] Having a loved one suspended midway between life and death is, however, for some families, a more desirable outcome than death. They cling desperately to that situation while awaiting a new medical breakthrough or a "miracle" that will restore the patient to a fully functioning status.

Talking to patients and their families is clearly a good way to resolve these conflicts. But what if, as in the case of Mrs. Wanglie, or Baby K,[33] or Mrs. Gilgunn, no amount of talking modifies or changes the opposing views? Rather than continue a fruitless attempt at ending an intractable dispute or going to court for a judicial determination on what should be done, the AMA's Council on Ethical and Judicial Affairs proposed that the best approach to resolve such conflicts is to implement a process that includes extensive deliberation and consultation followed by efforts to transfer care to a physician willing to comply with the patient (or family's) wishes.[34] If such a physician cannot be identified and the transfer affected, the attending physician may withhold or withdraw treatments deemed inappropriate.

The AMA's policy offers professional guidance, but it does not give legal protection to the physician. Such a legal "safe harbor," however, has been provided by recent legislation in both Texas[35] and California.[36] There if a physician has had broad consultation and offered the option of a transfer and the transfer cannot be arranged within ten days [or in California "it appears that a transfer cannot be accomplished"], the physician may cease interventions judged to be ineffective or inappropriate.

Fine and Mayo have analyzed the effectiveness of the Texas policy in resolving the kinds of conflicts we have been discussing.[37] They report that at Baylor Medical Center there was a 67 percent increase in the number of futility cases brought to the ethics committee after the legislation was enacted. Of the six cases in the Baylor study that were pursued through the dispute-resolution process, three families agreed to withdrawal of life-sustaining treatment within a few days of receiving a formal written report of the ethics committee. In two cases the patient died during the ten-day waiting period without an alternative provider having been found. In one case an alternative provider was located, but the patient died while awaiting transfer.

Though Texas law allowed it, no family member in the Baylor examples chose to challenge the judgment of the ethics consultation process in court. Fine and Mayo report that many families, even those who had vigorously opposed termination of treatment, seemed relieved by the process. As the authors summarized the issue, the families' position was "If you are asking us to agree with the recommendation to remove life support from our loved one, we cannot. However, if the law says it is OK to stop, then that is what should happen."[38]

Here the families are reflecting Dostoevsky's insight that individuals do not want the responsibility for such an awesome decision as ending the life of a loved one.[39] The ambiguity, anxiety, doubt, and guilt involved in such a decision are simply too much to bear. Rather they seek some authority to assume the decision-making role and thereby absolve them of the burden. If Dostoevsky is correct that the psychological trauma of having a family member, in effect, sign a death warrant before a death can occur is more burden than many individuals can sustain, then our insistence that patient autonomy requires that the patient or proxy "sign on the dotted line" before death can be allowed, may need to be revisited.

CONCLUSION

In a very early Picasso painting entitled "Science and Charity" the artist portrayed medicine as having two distinct roles: the delivery of scientific knowledge and the comfort of the patient. When the first is exhausted, as is true for the dying patient, the second remains a continuing task. The charity aspect is portrayed in the painting by a nun holding the patient's infant daughter in one arm while presenting the woman with a glass of water. Today, for better or worse, the nun is no longer in the picture. The "charity" aspect of medicine, however, continues as an ongoing challenge to both families as physicians. "Rage, rage against the fading light" does not seem to be an apt formula for fulfilling that role.

NOTES

1. The poem "Do Not Go Gentle Into That Good Night," by Dylan Thomas is reproduced from Dylan Thomas, *The Poems of Dylan Thomas* (New York: New Directions, 1952), 18. Copyright © 1952 by Dylan Thomas. Reprinted by permission of New Directions Publishing Corp.

2. Daniel Callahan, *The Troubled Dream of Life: Living with Mortality* (New York: Simon & Schuster, 1993).

3. Stanley J. Reiser, Arthur J. Dyck, and William J. Curran, eds., "Hippocratic Corpus: The Art," in *Ethics in Medicine: Historical Perspectives and Contemporary Concerns* (Cambridge, Mass.: MIT Press, 1977), 6–7.

4. Hippocrates, "The Art," in *Hippocrates*, trans. W. H. S. Jones (Cambridge, Mass.: Harvard University Press, 1923), 317–18.

5. Vatican, 1980 "Declaration on Euthanasia," reprinted in the President's Commission for the Study of Ethical Problems in Medicine and Biomedical

Research, *Deciding to Forego Life-Sustaining Treatment* (Washington, D.C.: Government Printing Office, 1983), 300–306.

6. Encyclical Letter *Evangelium Vitae* Addressed By The Supreme Pontiff Pope John Paul II To All The Bishops, Priests, And Deacons Men And Women Religious Lay Faithful And All People Of Good Will On The Value And Inviolability Of Human Life.

7. James J. McCartney, "The Development of the Doctrine of Ordinary and Extraordinary means of Preserving Life in Catholic Moral Theology before the Karen Quinlan Case," *Linacre Quarterly* 47 (1980): 215–26.

8. President's Commission, *Deciding to Forego Life-Sustaining Treatment*, 86–89.

9. Paul Ramsey, "On (Only) Caring for the Dying," in *The Patient As Person* (New Haven, Conn.: Yale University Press, 1970), 113–64.

10. Gerald Kelly, "The Duty of Using Artificial Means of Preserving Life," *Theological Studies* 12 (1950): 550–56.

11. Kelly, "The Duty of Using Artificial Means of Preserving Life," 556.

12. Richard A. McCormick, "To Save or Let Die: The Dilemma of Modern Medicine," *Journal of the American Medical Association* 229 (1974): 172–76.

13. Edmund D. Pellegrino, "The Metamorphosis of Medical Ethics: A Thirty Year Retrospective," *Journal of the American Medical Association* 269 (1993): 1158–62.

14. *Cruzan v. Director, Missouri Department of Health*, 497 U.S. 261, 110 S.Ct.2841(1990).

15. See, for example, Susan Wolf, "Near Death—In the Moment of Decision," *New England Journal of Medicine* 322 (1990): 208–10; and Robert M. Veatch and Carol M. Spicer, "Medical Futile Care: the Role of the Physician in Setting Limits," *American Journal of Law & Medicine* 18 (1992): 15–36.

16. Mary Harris, "Cost Conscious Hospitals Set Futile Care Rules." *American Medical News* (June 28, 1993): 1.

17. Stanley B. Fiel, "Heart-Lung Transplantation for Patients with Cystic-Fibrosis," *Archives of Internal Medicine* 151 (1991): 870–72.

18. Robert D. Truog, Alan S. Brett, and Joel Frader, "The Problem with Futility," *New England Journal of Medicine* 326 (1992): 1560–64.

19. Truog, Brett, and Frader, "The Problem With Futility."

20. Stewart J. Younger, "Who Defines Futility?" *Journal of the American Medical Association* 260 (1990): 2094–95.

21. John D. Lantos, Peter A. Singer, Robert M. Walker, et al., "The Illusion of Futility in Clinical Practice," *American Journal of Medicine* 87 (1989): 81–84.

22. Robert D. Truog, "Beyond Futility," *Journal of Clinical Ethics* 3 (1992): 143–45.

23. Lawrence J. Schneiderman, Kathy Faber-Langendoen, and Nancy S. Jecker, "Beyond Futility to an Ethics of Care," *Annals of Internal Medicine* 96 (1994): 110–14.

24. Younger, "Who Defines Futility?"

25. Lawrence J. Schneiderman, Nancy S. Jecker, and Albert R. Jonsen, "Medical Futility: Its Meaning and Ethical Implications," *Annals of Internal Medicine* 112 (1990): 949–54.

26. David Johnson, "Helga Wanglie Revisited: Medical Futility and the Limits of Autonomy," *Cambridge Quarterly of Healthcare Ethics* 2 (1993): 161–70.

27. Marcia Angell, "The Case of Helga Wanglie: A New Kind of Right to Die Case," *New England Journal of Medicine* 325 (1991): 511–12.

28. T. Tomlinson and H. Brody, "Ethics and Communication in Do-Not-Resuscitate Orders," *New England Journal of Medicine* 318 (1990): 43–46.

29. American College of Chest Physicians/Society for Critical Care Medicine Consensus Panel: "Ethical and Moral Guidelines for the Initiation, Continuation and Withdrawal of Intensive Care," *Chest* 97 (1990): 949–58; American Thoracic Society Bioethics Task Force: "Withholding and Withdrawing Life-Sustaining Therapy," Annals of Internal Medicine 115 (1991): 478–85; Emergency Cardiac Care Committee and Subcommittees, American Heart Association: "Guidelines for Cardiopulmonary Resuscitation and Emergency Cardiac Care: VIII. Ethical Considerations in Resuscitation," *Journal of the American Medical Association* 268 (1992): 2282–88; and Task Force on Ethics of the Society of Critical Care Medicine: "Consensus Report on the Ethics of Foregoing Life-Sustaining Treatments in the Critically Ill," *Critical Care Medicine* 18 (1990): 1435–39.

30. Paul Helft, Mark Siegler, and John Lantos, "The Rise and Fall of the Futility Movement," *New England Journal of Medicine*, July 27, 2000.

31. Stewart J. Younger, "Applying Futility: Saying No Is Not Enough," *Journal of The American Geriatric Society* 42 (1994): 887–89.

32. *In re Dinnerstein*, 380 N.E. 2d 134 (Mass. App. 1978).

33. "In the Matter of Baby K," 16 f3D 590 (4th Cir. 1994).

34. Council on Ethical and Judicial Affairs, American Medical Association, "Medical Futility in End-of-Life Care," *Journal of the American Medical Association* 281 (1991): 937–41.

35. Texas Health and Safety Code § 166.046 (2) (1999).

36. California Probate Code § 4736 (West. 2000).

37. Robert K. Fine and Thomas Wm. Mayo, "Resolution of Futility by Due Process: Early Experience with the Texas Advance Directive Act," *Annals of Internal Medicine* 138 (2003): 743–46.

38. Fine and Mayo, "Resolution of Futility by Due Process," 746.

39. John D. Lantos, "The Karamazov Complex: Dostoevsky and DNR Orders," *Perspectives in Biology & Medicine* 45 (2002): 190–99.

III

AFTER DEATH: RESPECT AND CULTURAL NORMS

8

Training on Newly Deceased Patients: An Ethical Analysis

Mark R. Wicclair

Medical procedures clearly cannot benefit the dead. Performing medical procedures on deceased patients, however, can directly benefit medical trainees and thereby indirectly benefit future patients. The use of newly deceased patients for medical training is quite common.[1] Practicing on dead humans is thought to have significant advantages over the alternatives. Using dead rather than living humans avoids any risk of morbidity or mortality. Using dead humans rather than nonhuman animals avoids the infliction of unnecessary pain and suffering on animals. Finally, practicing on dead humans rather than using mannequins and computer simulations is believed to provide a more effective means for medical trainees to acquire clinical skills.[2]

Yet even if these claims about the advantages of practicing on newly dead patients are warranted, the end does not always justify the means. This chapter discusses the ethical issues raised by this practice. It argues that training on newly deceased patients can be ethically permissible so long as appropriate respect is shown toward the deceased patients and their families. It also discusses the consent requirements that must be satisfied if appropriate respect is to be shown.

IS IT *PER SE* UNETHICAL TO
PRACTICE ON THE DEAD?

Are there reasons to think that practicing on the newly dead is *per se* unethical? It might be claimed that it is disrespectful to practice on the bodies of patients after they die. More dramatically, it might be objected that using dead patients' bodies in this way is indistinguishable from abusing or desecrating corpses. Although these claims should be taken seriously, it is important to see that they fail to establish that training on the dead is *per se* unethical. As the practices of autopsies, organ donation, and cremation demonstrate, the line between respectful and disrespectful treatment of corpses cannot be based exclusively on what is done to a body. Medical examiners, serial murderers, and terrorists dissect and dismember bodies. From the perspective of what is done to cadavers (i.e., what a video camera would capture), there is a similarity. By contrast, from the perspective of whether the corpses are treated disrespectfully—at least according to prevailing social norms in the United States—there is no similarity.

To be sure, standards of respectful treatment of corpses can vary considerably from culture to culture and from person to person.[3] For example, even practices that are widely accepted in the United States, such as autopsies and cremation, are viewed as "disrespectful" by some groups. Accordingly, training on the dead may be viewed as disrespectful according to one set of cultural and/or religious norms, but not another. Consequently, it is unwarranted to assert that performing medical procedures on newly deceased patients for training purposes is *per se* disrespectful of the dead. Indeed, the primary ethical controversy in relation to training on newly deceased patients assumes that doing so is not *per se* disrespectful and focuses on the question: Is consent to practice on the newly deceased ethically required?[4]

PREMORTEM CONSENT

Obviously, the deceased patient cannot give or refuse consent, but it is possible to give patients an opportunity to consent or refuse while they are still alive. The importance of premortem consent or refusal is already recognized by the Uniform Anatomical Gift Act (UAGA), which is the model for legislation in all states.[5] That act authorizes people to give or withhold consent to use their bodies or specified parts of their bodies "for transplantation, therapy, medical or dental *education*, research, or advancement of medical or dental science" after death.[6]

There are several reasons why it is ethically desirable, when feasible, to give individuals an opportunity to give or withhold consent to training on their bodies after death. One reason derives from the commonly recognized right to control what happens in and to one's body. This right can be conceptualized as a liberty or privacy right or a property right, and it can be justified by appealing to a number of different foundational ethical theories, including consequentialism, contractarianism, and rights-based theories.[7] Intuitively, it can be said to derive from the inseparability of a person and his or her body: events and actions that affect my body *ipso facto* affect *me*. To be sure, when a person dies, the person ceases to exist, but the body does not. In this respect, then, the person and his or her body are no longer inseparable after death. However, it still is the case that there is one and only one living person with whom a particular body had a unique and inseparable relationship. Accordingly, it might be claimed that this distinctive relationship, and the enduring association between the body and the person whose body it was, provide sufficient reason to extend a right to control what happens in and to one's body after death.

Generally, regardless of the preferred justification of the right to control what happens in and to one's body, a justification of the same type can be used to support giving people control over the treatment of their bodies after death. For example, if utilitarian, contractarian, or rights-based reasons are given to support the claim that I have a right today to refuse access to my body by physicians and trainees tomorrow if I am alive, reasons of the same type can be given to assert that I have a right today to refuse access to my body by physicians and trainees tomorrow if I am dead. However, even if the same *type* of justification can be given for a right to control what happens in and to one's body before and after death, specific appeals may differ. For example, whereas a justification of a right to control what happens in and to one's body *before* death might cite the experiences of a person following an unwanted invasion of his or her body, a justification of a right to control what happens in and to one's body *after* death could cite only (anticipatory) premortem experiences—e.g., the repulsion a person might feel at the thought of his or her body being used for training after death. In addition, there may be reasons for overriding the right after death that do not apply, or are insufficient, prior to death—e.g., determining whether a person's death was the result of a criminal act—and reasons that are sufficient to override the right after death may not be sufficient prior to death.

As important as it may be ethically to give people an opportunity to decide in advance whether or not to give their permission to use their bodies for training after death, studies of organ donation suggest the limits of this practice. According to a 1993 Gallup Organization survey, although 69 percent of respondents stated that they were either "very likely" (37 percent) or "somewhat likely" (32 percent) to want to have their organs donated after death, only 42 percent reported already having decided whether or not to donate.[8] Moreover, despite the fact that only 25 percent of the respondents stated that they were either "not very likely" or "not at all likely" to want to have their organs donated after death, only 55 percent stated that they either already had a donor card (28 percent), or would be willing to get one (27 percent). These results suggest that people who are reluctant to give advance consent are not necessarily opposed to becoming organ donors after death.

A study of people who had been asked to donate the organs of deceased family members suggests two reasons why individuals who are not opposed in principle to donating their organs after death may be reluctant to make and document such a decision before death. First, individuals fear that providing premortem consent might have a negative impact on the medical care they receive. And second, they desire family members to have a role in deciding whether or not to donate their organs.[9] If these results are generalizable, then when the living are given an opportunity to decide in advance whether to authorize using their bodies for training after they die, they should be presented with the following range of choices: (1) to give (restricted or unrestricted) permission; (2) to refuse permission; (3) to indicate a preference that others—e.g., family—decide after the individual's death; or (4) to indicate that the individual does not want to make any decision at the current time.[10]

SURROGATE (FAMILY) CONSENT

When deceased patients have not decided prior to death whether to allow training on their bodies after they die, consent should be sought from an appropriate surrogate. Surviving family members are presumptively considered appropriate surrogates since they are most likely to be familiar with the deceased's premortem preferences and values and since family members have a legitimate interest in protecting the deceased's remains. This presumption has legal support. Family members generally are legally responsible for the disposition of corpses;[11] and according to the UAGA, the only people authorized to make anatomical gifts, other than the donor and the deceased's guardian, are family members in the following order of priority: a spouse, an adult son or daughter, an adult brother or sister, and a grandparent.[12]

Respect for the Dead

There are several reasons for requiring family consent. One of the most important among them is that requiring family consent can promote respect for the dead by fostering respect for the deceased's premortem preferences and values. On the one hand, in the absence of direct evidence concerning the deceased patient's preferences, allowing the family to decide is the next best means to respect any preferences that the deceased may have had about the use and disposition of his or her body. On the other hand, if the deceased did not document such preferences prior to death, it is reasonable to presume that he or she would have wanted family members to decide about the use and disposition of the body. One study reported that 71 percent of respondents indicated that they agreed or strongly agreed with the proposition that they would want family members to be asked for permission to practice lifesaving skills on their bodies after they died.[13]

But why should the premortem preferences of dead patients matter ethically? It might be conceded that people's premortem *decisions* concerning whether or not their bodies may be used for clinical training after death should be honored out of respect for the rights of the living. That is, it might be acknowledged that people have a right, while alive, to execute a directive (an "advance refusal") that has moral (and legal) force after death and which records a refusal to allow trainees to practice procedures on their corpses. However, one might claim that in the absence of such a documented *decision*, it is not ethically required to consider premortem preferences and values. Kenneth Iserson presents a view along these lines.[14] In defense of practicing medical procedures on the dead without securing the permission of family members, he asserts: "Simple as the concept is, corpses no longer are individuals, and so they cannot be the basis for either autonomy or informed consent. They are merely symbols."[15]

To be sure, corpses no longer are *living* individuals, but they can be individuated as the body (or body parts) of a particular person. Why is it that corpses "cannot be the basis for either autonomy or informed consent"? Is it, perhaps, because nothing matters to the dead? Or, is it because the dead are "no longer persons"?[16] The first reason would apply to people who are permanently unconscious, and, depending on one's criteria of "personhood," the second reason also might apply to people who are permanently unconscious as well as to people with advanced dementia. Yet, a recognized standard of surrogate decision making—one that applies to all decisionally incapacitated patients who previously had decision-making capacity, including the permanently unconscious and severely demented individuals—is "substituted judgment," which instructs surrogates to consider the patient's prior preferences and values.[17]

As the accepted practice of honoring people's premortem preferences and values in relation to organ donation and burial indicates, it is generally acknowledged that such preferences and values warrant respect. But, it might still be asked, what is the ethical basis for respecting premortem preferences of the dead? One ethical basis is respect for (living) persons. It might reasonably be claimed that it would be incompatible with respect for persons if, at the moment of death, we were to abruptly cease attributing moral force to any of a deceased's premortem preferences and values. To show respect for a person is to acknowledge his or her worth, dignity, and autonomy; and it can be said that we would fail to show such respect if we were to believe and act as if an individual's distinctive aspirations, plans, and preferences left no "moral traces" after death.

A second ethical basis for respecting premortem preferences and values after death is that it can contribute to the well-being of the living. Generally, the belief that all of one's preferences and values will not simply be disregarded after one's death can be a source of considerable reassurance and comfort while one is alive. Conversely, the belief that one's preferences and values will be given no moral weight after one's death can be a source of considerable anxiety, anguish, and distress. In addition, by continuing to respect premortem preferences and values after death, survivors give expression to the view that death does not signify a total annihilation of any "traces" of the person who once was. The person may be dead, but traces survive insofar as the living do not completely disregard premortem preferences and values. The resulting sense that some of one's preferences and values will continue to matter to the living after one dies may be important to people as they contemplate their own deaths, and there can be a corresponding impact on the well-being of survivors. To be sure, this "survival" of premortem preferences and values is not immortality, but it may give some solace to believe that such traces of ourselves will survive in the moral conceptions and actions of others.

Requiring family consent can also promote respect for the dead by preventing the deceased's body from being subject to undignified treatment (e.g., abuse of a corpse). It is generally acknowledged that human corpses should be treated with respect. The commitment to this principle was confirmed by the general condemnation of a crematory in Noble, Georgia, that dumped bodies slated for cremation on the facility's grounds, where they were discovered later in various stages of decomposition.[18] More recently, a scandal involving the Willed Body Program at the University of California, Los Angeles, generated a series of articles in the *New York Times*, one of which appeared to assume that readers would be disturbed to learn that corpses were "mangled in automobile crash tests, blown to bits by land mines, or cut up with power saws to be shipped in pieces around the country or even abroad."[19]

As already noted, there is considerable variation in standards of respectful treatment of corpses. Accordingly, an appropriate aim is to avoid treating a corpse in a way that *the deceased person* would have considered disrespectful. The deceased's family may well be in the best position to determine whether using the body for training is consistent with the deceased patient's conception of respect for corpses. But even if the deceased's conception is unknown, it seems appropriate for the family to act as the deceased's representative for the purpose of determining whether postmortem training is compatible with respect for human corpses, just as it is generally appropriate for family members to act as surrogates for patients in clinical contexts even when it is impossible to make accurate substituted judgments. Significantly, the law recognizes the role of family members in determining what consti-

tutes "abuse of corpses." For example, the section of the Model Penal
Code entitled "Abuse of Corpse" states: "Except as authorized by law,
a person who treats a corpse in a way that he knows would *outrage
ordinary family sensibilities* commits a misdemeanor."[20]

Respect for the Family

Requiring family consent also shows respect for grieving family members. Family members are likely to perceive a significant continuity
between the person who died and the dead body. Such an association
between living persons and dead bodies is to be expected since we
encounter other persons—and to some extent even ourselves—via the
body (its distinctive appearance, movements, sounds, smells, and so
forth). Indeed, it might be said that the body is the best (only) physical
representation of the person or self. Accordingly, family members may
want to decide whether to authorize training on the bodies of their dead
loved ones, just as they often want to decide whether to authorize medical interventions for decisionally incapacitated relatives. One study
reported that, depending on the procedure, between 73.8 percent and
87.2 percent of relatives of patients being evaluated in an emergency
department would want to be asked for their consent if the patient were
to die and physicians proposed to practice procedures on the deceased's
body.[21] Significantly, depending on the procedure, between 53 percent
and 73.7 percent of the relatives reported that they would consent. Both
conclusions are supported by at least one other study.[22] Thus, wanting
to be asked is *not* correlated with a predisposition to refuse.

A perceived continuity between the living person and the dead body
may prompt family members to associate care for the body with care
for the dead loved one. For example, one study reported that a common
reason given by family members of newly deceased patients for refusing consent to retrograde tracheal intubation for research purposes was
that the patient "had suffered enough."[23] In another study, approximately 25 percent of relatives of newly deceased patients who refused
consent for teaching intubation cited a desire "to leave the dead in
peace."[24] A study of consent for teaching intubation skills on newly
deceased infants reported that among families who refused consent,
"the common theme was 'No, our baby has been through enough.'"[25]
Even if such beliefs were to mistakenly assume that the dead can suffer

and experience discomfort, it would be incompatible with respect for grieving families—and insensitive—to dismiss their wishes on the grounds that they have an "irrational" basis.

In addition, family members might well experience considerable emotional distress if they were to witness unconsented use of a loved one's body for training or if they were to discover after the fact that medical procedures were practiced without consent on a dead loved one. One study reported that 60 percent of respondents would be "upset" if procedures were practiced on their bodies without consent and 50 percent would have a similar response if procedures were practiced on the bodies of relatives without prior consent.[26] Surely, it is desirable to prevent grieving families from experiencing avoidable harms. Harm aside, even if it were feasible to prevent families from discovering that their loved ones' bodies were used to practice medical procedures, a need to conceal would fail the "transparency" test and therefore would be morally suspect.

Finally, seeking the permission of family members expresses respect for the family as a valued social institution by recognizing a zone of *family* privacy and autonomy.[27]

Fostering an Educational Environment that Nurtures Ethical Sensitivity

Medical trainees have expressed discomfort about practicing procedures on newly deceased patients, especially without consent.[28] A study of parents' willingness to consent to practicing intubation on newly deceased infants included the following comment by a resident: "As long as parents agree to allow intubation, I feel comfortable about doing it. Once, as a medical student we practiced on a deceased patient without family permission, and I felt very uncomfortable doing it."[29] Indeed, it was a medical student initiative that led the Council on Ethical and Judicial Affairs (CEJA) of the American Medical Association (AMA) to consider whether consent should be required for training on newly deceased patients.[30] The resulting CEJA report[31] was the basis for Opinion 8.181, "Performing Procedures on the Newly Deceased,"[32] which requires consent. Such trainee unease reflects a legitimate concern for the dignity of deceased patients and the interests and emotional well-being of grieving family members. If ethically sensitive trainees are uncomfortable practicing on newly deceased patients without family consent, they should not be encouraged to "overcome" that discomfort. Quite the contrary, ethical sensitivity on the part of trainees should be reinforced and nurtured.

Like family members, health care professionals and trainees may perceive a continuity between a person and that person's body after death.[33] To undermine this perception by encouraging trainees to ignore the connection between a cadaver and the patient for whom they previously cared might adversely affect the way in which trainees perceive live patients (i.e., as mere bodies rather than embodied *persons*). A similar concern has been expressed in relation to the impact of dissection of cadavers on medical students. Several strategies have been employed within the context of anatomy courses to prevent desensitization and depersonalization and to promote instead humanistic attitudes toward patient care.[34]

Trust

A failure to request the consent of family may undermine public trust in the medical profession.[35] Keeping family members "out of the loop" is likely to engender suspicion and mistrust. This holds true no matter how "benign" the reasons are for not seeking consent. Such suspicion and mistrust may undermine the physician-patient relationship and may diminish the willingness of people to make anatomical gifts. The importance of trust also provides a further reason for insisting on transparency in the process of practicing on newly deceased patients.

CONFLICTS BETWEEN PREMORTEM CONSENT AND FAMILY WISHES

Prior to death, individuals have an ethical and legal right to decide to make anatomical gifts. The primary ethical basis is autonomy and the primary legal basis is the UAGA. The UAGA specifically states that family members have no legal authority to override an anatomical gift after the donor's death: "An anatomical gift that is not revoked by the donor before death is irrevocable and does not require the consent or concurrence of any person after the donor's death."[36] This view can be justified ethically by claiming that the autonomy rights of the person whose body is at issue trump the autonomy rights of family members. Moreover, there is some anecdotal evidence that family members who initially opposed honoring the premortem decisions of loved ones to become organ donors later come to accept the decision to retrieve organs despite their initial objections.[37]

It is reasonable to assume that people who have "organ donor" designations on their driver's licenses or who carry organ donor cards intended to donate organs for transplantation. However, depending on the state, people may not be aware that, in addition to transplantation, the terms "organ donor" and "anatomical gift" under the UAGA include use for education unless the donor has explicitly indicated otherwise. Thus, although premortem *consent* for postmortem education and training trumps family wishes to the contrary, possession of an organ donor card is not necessarily evidence of premortem *informed consent* for education and training.

To recognize the ethical significance of premortem decisions to make anatomical gifts, it is reasonable to adopt a *rebuttable presumption* that an organ donor card or driver's license with an "organ donor" designation authorizes education and training as well as organ donation despite family objections. To acknowledge the value of family decision making, the legitimate interests of surviving relatives, and the ambiguity of donor documents concerning donor intent, it is reasonable to permit family members to rebut this presumption by providing evidence to support the conclusion that although the decedent wanted organs to be used for transplant, he or she would not have wanted the body to be used for education.

When training is to be undertaken with the authorization of a donor card, family members need not be asked for their *permission*, but they at least should be *informed* before any procedures are performed. Informing family members gives them an opportunity to object, and the basis of their objection can then be explored. If there are any doubts about the donor's intent, it is appropriate to ask family members whether they have any reason to believe that although the decedent decided to be an organ donor, he would not have wanted his body used for training. Optimally, a discussion of the intentions of the donor will take place prior to death and, unless the donor objects, the family will be present.

OBJECTIONS TO A CONSENT REQUIREMENT

Prior to the adoption by the AMA House of Delegates in 2001 of the policy endorsing a consent requirement, it was common to train on newly deceased patients without consent.[38] The common practice of training without consent suggests a belief that consent is not ethically required. What reasons can be given to support this belief?

The view that the living have an ethical and legal right to decide whether or not to permit their bodies to be used for training after death is hardly subject to serious challenge. Accordingly, challenges to a consent requirement generally take the form of denying the need for family consent when deceased patients did not decide to give or withhold consent prior to death. One of these challenges takes the form of disputing an alleged goal of a family consent requirement: respect for the deceased's premortem preferences and values.[39] This objection was critically examined above. Additional challenges to a family consent requirement include the following: (1) it will result in a significant reduction in opportunities to practice medical procedures, (2) it will add to the distress and emotional trauma of grieving families, (3) consent is not required when procedures are minimally invasive and involve no disfigurement of the corpse, and (4) consent is not required when trainees perform procedures on living patients.

A Significant Reduction in Opportunities to Practice Medical Procedures

One reason for thinking that a family consent requirement will substantially reduce opportunities to practice medical procedures on the dead is the belief that if asked, most families will decline permission. This belief rests on the assumption that grieving families immediately after the death of a loved one are not likely to authorize postmortem training. However, the available evidence does not support such an assumption. One study reported that when permission was requested from forty-three families to perform a cricothyrotomy on a newly deceased relative, twenty (47 percent) consented.[40] Another study reported that when forty-four parents of infants who died in a neonatal intensive care unit were asked to allow intubation for teaching purposes, thirty-two (73 percent) consented.[41] Two larger studies reported that the vast majority of family members would be willing to consent to practicing procedures on a deceased relative's body.[42]

A second reason for thinking that a family consent requirement will substantially reduce opportunities to practice medical procedures on the dead is the belief that attending physicians and trainees will be reluctant to ask permission from grieving family members. For example, Iserson claims that faced with a family consent requirement, clinicians might decide to forgo practicing on the dead because "[t]he need to request . . . permission from distraught relatives would raise significant emotional barriers for clinicians to overcome in order to practice and teach the procedures."[43] However, if there are valid ethical reasons for requiring family consent, then clinician training should include efforts to overcome these barriers and facilitate communication with families of deceased patients.[44] Alternatively, using organ procurement as a model, the responsibility for seeking consent might be assigned to specially trained personnel, such as organ procurement organization (OPO) representatives.

Finally, it might be objected that there may be substantial practical hurdles, such as time constraints and/or unavailability of family members, which prevent always asking families for consent. In response, it can be held that in such cases, unless the deceased patient consented prior to death, it would be ethically unacceptable to proceed without family permission. Although the UAGA permits a qualified exception to the consent requirement, that exception is limited to transplant and therapy, which reflects a judgment about the special importance of measures that can directly save lives. CEJA Opinion 8.181, "Performing Procedures on the Newly Deceased," also allows no exception to the consent requirement in relation to training: "When reasonable efforts to discover previously expressed preferences of the deceased or to find someone with authority to grant permission for the procedure have failed, physicians must not perform procedures for training purposes on the newly deceased patient."[45]

The foregoing reasons to reject a consent requirement are not only unpersuasive, but also incomplete. For even if it were the case that requiring consent would result in fewer opportunities to practice on the dead than if consent were not required, it would remain to show that there are no satisfactory alternatives to training on recently deceased patients and that the value of the increase in opportunities to practice on the dead outweighs the ethical importance of obtaining consent. However, studies comparing the effectiveness of different teaching models are limited in size and scope;[46] and there is insufficient empirical evidence to establish how many and what kind of opportunities to train, if any, would be lost if a consent requirement were adopted. Moreover, weighing the importance of training vs. consent may require controversial value judgments. To maintain that an interest in practicing procedures on the dead generally trumps consent would be contrary to the prevailing view in the United States in relation to retrieving organs for transplant, where there is a documented shortage and where the expected benefit is arguably both more certain and immediate than that of training on recently deceased patients. As noted above, the UAGA allows only a limited exception to the requirement of donor or surrogate consent, one that applies only to transplantation or therapy, and not to education.[47]

Adding to the Distress of Grieving Families

A second reason for rejecting a consent requirement is the alleged negative impact on grieving family members.[48] At a time when they are already emotionally overwrought, it is claimed, it would be insensitive to burden them with an upsetting decision. As emphasized above, respect for grieving family members and concern for their emotional well-being are important. However, it is crucial not to confuse concern for the emotional well-being of grieving family members with the discomfort of *trainees*, which stems in part from a reluctance to discuss death with family members.[49] Benfield and colleagues speculate that "self-protection" may play a role: "Perhaps then, intubating newly dead adults without consent is done not only to protect family emotions but also to protect some physicians from emotional discomfort and the possibility of being refused."[50] In addition, the experience in relation to organ transplantation suggests that requesting consent may not have a predominantly negative impact on the deceased's family. Studies report that family members appreciate having been given an opportunity to donate a loved one's organs and that donation can lessen grief.[51] For many it can provide some comfort and meaning in a context of loss and senselessness, and a similar benefit may be associated with consent for training.[52] This may well be a situation in which paternalism is not only unwarranted, but counterproductive as well. Significantly, one study about requests for training on newly deceased patients reported that only one of thirty-two families who were asked for permission to perform a cricothyrotomy on a recently deceased patient stated six weeks later that they were "offended or upset about being approached for the procedure."[53]

Procedures are Minimally Invasive and Involve No Disfigurement of the Corpse

A third objection to a family consent requirement points out that many of the procedures that are practiced on newly deceased patients are minimally invasive and involve no disfigurement of the corpse.[54] Accordingly, it is claimed, there is no need to request permission from family members. Yet whether or not procedures are invasive or disfiguring, asking for consent still expresses respect for the deceased and family members. Moreover, even if there are no physical marks, training on newly deceased patients can violate the deceased's and/or the deceased's family's conception of dignity and/or respectful treatment of corpses. The absence of physical marks may make it possible to perform procedures without detection by family members. However, such violations of transparency threaten public trust and are ethically unacceptable.

Consent is Not Required When Trainees Perform Procedures on Living Patients

A fourth reason for rejecting a family consent requirement is based on the observation that *living patients* often are not asked for their permission when trainees perform medical procedures. Accordingly, it is objected that requiring consent for training in the case of deceased patients would apply a stricter standard to the dead than to living patients. As Orlowski puts it: "It would be ironic if these institutions [i.e., hospitals] required consent to practice procedures on cadavers, but permitted students and residents to practice and learn procedures on living patients without expressed, informed consent for each procedure and each occurrence."[55]

To assess this objection, there is no need to determine whether it is ethically justified for trainees to perform medical procedures on living patients without their explicit informed consent. For even if informed consent is not always ethically required in such contexts, there are significant differences between training on living and deceased patients. First, with the exception of emergent situations, although consent may not be sought for allowing a *trainee* rather than an attending physician to perform a clinically indicated procedure, consent *is* sought for *the procedure*. Second, although performing such procedures may also contribute to a trainee's acquisition of clinical skills, an important goal is to benefit the patient. By contrast, procedures cannot benefit deceased patients, and training is the exclusive goal. Hence, the practice of not requiring a patient's consent to having a *trainee*, rather than an attending physician, perform a clinically indicated procedure fails to provide a suitable analogue for not requiring consent when trainees perform procedures on newly deceased patients.

CONCLUSION

This chapter has argued that while it is not *per se* unethical to perform medical procedures on newly deceased patients for training purposes, this practice does raise important ethical concerns. To be ethically acceptable, training on newly deceased patients must be respectful of deceased patients as well as their families. Respect for deceased patients requires honoring any premortem decisions they might have made about using their bodies for training. It also requires respecting their premortem preferences, if they are known.

When deceased patients have not decided prior to death whether to allow their bodies to be used for training, respect for them and their families generally requires the consent of family members. The available evidence suggests that a consent requirement will neither impose a substantial obstacle to practicing on newly deceased patients nor significantly increase the emotional distress of grieving families. A family consent requirement also serves to foster an educational environment for trainees that nurtures ethical sensitivity, promotes public trust in the medical profession, and sustains compliance with the Uniform Anatomical Gift Act (UAGA) and statutes that prohibit abuse of corpses.

NOTES

1. Council on Ethical and Judicial Affairs of the American Medical Association, "Performing Procedures on the Newly Deceased," *Academic Medicine* 77, no. 12 (2002): 212–16.

2. Andrew W. Alden, Kristen L. M. Ward, and Gregory P. Moore, "Should Postmortem Procedures Be Practiced on Recently Deceased Patients? A Survey of Relatives' Attitudes," *Academic Emergency Medicine* 6, no. 7 (1999): 749–52; and James P. Orlowski, George A. Kanoti, and Maxwell J. Mehlman, "The Ethical Dilemma of Permitting the Teaching and Perfecting of Resuscitation Techniques on Recently Expired Patients," *Journal of Clinical Ethics* 1, no. 3 (1990): 201–5.

3. Peter Metcalf and Richard Huntington, *Celebrations of Death*, 2nd ed. (Cambridge: Cambridge University Press, 1991).

4. Council on Ethical and Judicial Affairs of the American Medical Association, "Performing Procedures on the Newly Deceased."

5. National Conference of Commissioners on Uniform State Laws, "Uniform Anatomical Gift Act," (1987).

6. National Conference of Commissioners on Uniform State Laws, "Uniform Anatomical Gift Act," Sec. 2a and 6a, emphasis added.

7. For a discussion of privacy and property conceptions of bodily autonomy, see Radhika Rao, "Property, Privacy, and the Human Body," *Boston University Law Review* 80 (2000): 359–460. For a discussion of various foundational ethical theories, see Shelly Kagan, *Normative Ethics* (Boulder, Colo.: Westview Press, 1998), part II.

8. Gallup Organization Inc., "The American Public's Attitudes toward Organ Donation and Transplantation" (Boston: The Partnership for Organ Donation, 1993).

9. See Laura A. Siminoff and Mary Beth Mercer, "Public Policy, Public Opinion, and Consent for Organ Donation," *Cambridge Quarterly of Healthcare Ethics* 10 (2001): 377–86.

10. Recognizing the drawbacks associated with mandated choice, Hayes proposes a modified form of mandated choice that would allow patients to decide not to decide. Gregory J. Hayes, "Issues of Consent: The Use of the Recently Deceased for Endotracheal Intubation Training," *Journal of Clinical Ethics* 5, no. 3 (1994): 211–16.

11. Tanya K. Hernandez, "The Property of Death," *University of Pittsburgh Law Review* 60 (1999): 971–1028; and Rao, "Property, Privacy, and the Human Body."

12. National Conference of Commissioners on Uniform State Laws, "Uniform Anatomical Gift Act," Section 3.

13. Kathleen S. Oman, John David Armstrong, II, and Martha Stoner, "Perspectives on Practicing Procedures on the Newly Dead," *Academic Emergency Medicine* 9, no. 8 (2002): 786–90.

14. Kenneth V. Iserson, "Life Versus Death: Exposing a Misapplication of Ethical Reasoning," *Journal of Clinical Ethics* 5 (1994): 261–66.

15. Iserson, "Life Versus Death," 262.

16. Kenneth V. Iserson, "Requiring Consent to Practice and Teach Using the Recently Dead," *Journal of Emergency Medicine* 9, no. 6 (1991): 509.

17. In the case of severely demented patients, there can be (perceived) conflicts between the patient's prior preferences and values and current (experiential) interests. See, for example, Rebecca Dresser, "Life, Death, and Incompetent Patients: Conceptual Infirmities and Hidden Values in the Law," *Arizona Law Review* 28 (1986): 373–405; and John A. Robertson, "Second Thoughts on Living Wills," *Hastings Center Report* 21, no. 6 (1991): 6–9. Obviously, there can be no such conflict in the case of the dead.

18. David Firestone and Robert D. McFadden, "Scores of Bodies Strewn at Site of Crematory," *New York Times*, February 17, 2002, 1, 25.

19. John M. Broder, "In Science's Name, Lucrative Trade in Body Parts," *New York Times*, March 12, 2004, 1, 19.

20. Model Penal Code, § 250.10 (2001); emphasis added.

21. Alden, Ward, and Moore, "Should Postmortem Procedures Be Practiced on Recently Deceased Patients?"

22. Sapal Tachakra, Selwyn Ho, Maria Lynch, and Roger Newson, "Should Doctors Practise Resuscitation Skills on Newly Deceased Patients? A Survey of Public Opinion," *Journal of the Royal Society of Medicine* 91, no. 11 (1998): 576–78.

23. Robert M. McNamara, Susan Monti, and John J. Kelly, "Requesting Consent for an Invasive Procedure in Newly Deceased Adults," *Journal of the American Medical Association* 273, no. 4 (1995): 310–12.

24. Guttorm Brattebo, Torben Wisborg, Kaare Solheim, and Nina Oyen, "Public Opinion on Different Approaches to Teaching Intubation Techniques," *British Medical Journal* 307, no. 6914 (1993): 1256–57.

25. D. Gary Benfield et al., "Teaching Intubation Skills Using Newly Deceased Infants," *Journal of the American Medical Association* 265, no. 18 (1991): 2362.

26. Craig A. Manifold, Alan Storrow, and Kevin Rodgers, "Patient and Family Attitudes Regarding the Practice of Procedures on the Newly Deceased," *Academic Emergency Medicine* 6, no. 2 (1999): 110–15.

27. Mark R. Wicclair, *Ethics and the Elderly* (New York: Oxford University Press, 1993), chapter 2.

28. Benfield et al., "Teaching Intubation Skills Using Newly Deceased Infants"; and Dan K. Morhaim and Michael B. Heller, "The Practice of Teaching Endotracheal Intubation on Recently Deceased Patients," *Journal of Emergency Medicine* 9 (1991): 515–18.

29. Benfield et al., "Teaching Intubation Skills Using Newly Deceased Infants," 2362.

30. A resolution introduced by the Medical Student Section during the AMA's

House of Delegates Interim Meeting in 2000 (I–00) requested that: "[The] American Medical Association study the issue of using deceased patients for training or other educational purposes and develop ethical guidelines regarding this practice." Resolution 1, I–00, "Requesting Consent for Invasive Procedures in the Newly Deceased Patient," *Proceedings of the American Medical Association's 2000 Interim Meeting of the House of Delegates*. See also Council on Ethical and Judicial Affairs of the American Medical Association, "Performing Procedures on the Newly Deceased."

31. Council on Ethical and Judicial Affairs of the American Medical Association, "Performing Procedures on the Newly Deceased."

32. Council on Ethical and Judicial Affairs of the American Medical Association, *Code of Medical Ethics: Current Opinions with Annotations*, 2002–2003 ed. (Chicago: AMA Press, 2002).

33. See, for example, Benfield et al., "Teaching Intubation Skills Using Newly Deceased Infants."

34. See, for example, Sandra L. Bertman and S. C. Marks Jr., "Humanities in Medical Education: Rationale and Resources for the Dissection Laboratory," *Medical Education* 19 (1985): 374–81; J. L. Coulehan, P. C. Williams, D. Landis, and C. Naser, "The First Patient: Reflections and Stories About the Anatomy Cadaver," *Teaching and Learning in Medicine* 7 (1995): 61–66; and Lawrence J. Rizzolo, "Human Dissection: An Approach to Interweaving the Traditional and Humanistic Goals of Medical Education," *The Anatomical Record (New Anat.)* 269 (2002): 242–48.

35. Jeffrey P. Burns, Frank E. Reardon, and Robert D. Truog, "Using Newly Deceased Patients to Teach Resuscitation Procedures," *New England Journal of Medicine* 331, no. 24 (1994): 1652–55.

36. National Conference of Commissioners on Uniform State Laws, "Uniform Anatomical Gift Act," Section 2(h).

37. Karen Sokohl, "First Person Consent," *UNOS Update* (2002): 2–3.

38. Mark W. Fourre, "The Performance of Procedures on the Recently Deceased," *Academic Emergency Medicine* 9, no. 6 (2002): 595–98; and Christopher J. Denny and Daniel Kollek, "Practicing Procedures on the Recently Dead," *Journal of Emergency Medicine* 17, no. 6 (1999): 949–52.

39. Iserson, "Life Versus Death."

40. Jon Olsen, Steve Spilger, and Tammy Windisch, "Feasibility of Obtaining Family Consent for Teaching Cricothyrotomy on the Newly Dead in the Emergency Department," *Annals of Emergency Medicine* 25, no. 5 (1995): 660–65.

41. Benfield et al., "Teaching Intubation Skills Using Newly Deceased Infants."

42. Alden, Ward, and Moore, "Should Postmortem Procedures Be Practiced on Recently Deceased Patients?"; and Manifold, Storrow, and Rodgers, "Patient and Family Attitudes Regarding the Practice of Procedures on the Newly Deceased."

43. Iserson, "Life Versus Death," 509.

44. Jon C. Olsen, Michael L. Buenefe, and William D. Falco, "Death in the

Emergency Department," *Annals of Emergency Medicine* 31, no. 6 (1998): 758–65.

45. Council on Ethical and Judicial Affairs of the American Medical Association, *Code of Medical Ethics.*

46. Jon Rosenson, Jeffrey A. Tabas, and Pat Patterson, "Teaching Invasive Procedures to Medical Students," *Journal of the American Medical Association* 291, no. 1 (2004): 119–20.

47. National Conference of Commissioners on Uniform State Laws, "Uniform Anatomical Gift Act," Section 4.

48. Kenneth V. Iserson, "Postmortem Procedures in the Emergency Department: Using the Recently Dead to Practice and Teach," *Journal of Medical Ethics* 19, no. 2 (1993): 92–98; and Iserson, "Life Versus Death."

49. Olsen, Spilger, and Windisch, "Feasibility of Obtaining Family Consent for Teaching Cricothyrotomy on the Newly Dead in the Emergency Department."

50. Benfield et al., "Teaching Intubation Skills Using Newly Deceased Infants." 2363.

51. Marilyn Rossman Bartucci and Peggy Rickard Bishop, "The Meaning of Organ Donation to Donor Families," *Anna Journal* 15, no. 6 (1987): 369–71, 410; Linda Phillips Riley and Margaret Beatty Coolican, "Needs of Families of Organ Donors: Facing Death and Life," *Critical Care Nurse* 19, no. 2 (1999): 53–59; and P. R. Rivers, S. M. Buse, B. A. Bivins, and H. M. Horst, "Organ and Tissue Procurement in the Acute Care Setting: Principles and Practice—Part 1," *Annals of Emergency Medicine* 19, no. 1 (1990): 78–85.

52. Orlowski, Kanoti, and Mehlman, "The Ethical Dilemma of Permitting the Teaching and Perfecting of Resuscitation Techniques on Recently Expired Patients."

53. Olsen, Spilger, and Windisch, "Feasibility of Obtaining Family Consent for Teaching Cricothyrotomy on the Newly Dead in the Emergency Department," 662.

54. Kenneth V. Iserson, "Law Versus Life: The Ethical Imperative to Practice and Teach Using the Newly Dead Emergency Department Patient," *Annals of Emergency Medicine* 25, no. 1 (1995): 91–94; and Iserson, "Postmortem Procedures in the Emergency Department."

55. James P. Orlowski, "Politically Correct Ethical Thinking and Intubation Practice on Cadavers," *Journal of Clinical Ethics* 5, no. 3 (1994): 257.

Appendix: Abstracts of the Chapters

Chapter One

Is death bad? If so, for whom is it bad, and wherein does its badness consist? These philosophical questions are largely ignored in contemporary medical education. This chapter argues that philosophical reflection on the badness of death can be relevant to good clinical practice. After reviewing the arguments of a number of important philosophers, it argues that the recognition that life has a natural limit can temper the tendency to overtreat dying patients. The chapter also argues that attention to the reasons why death is bad, and for whom it is bad, can help clinicians from running together the badness for them of the death of their patients with the badness of death for the patients who are dying.

Chapter Two

Recent advances in medical technology have complicated the question of when patients die. This chapter surveys the controversy over defining death, identifying a number of key areas of disagreement. It then proposes and defends the whole-brain formulation of the brain-death criterion. The chapter argues that an adequate criterion of death must square with our ordinary consensual usage of the concept and that the whole-brain formulation fares well along this dimension.

Chapter Three

Should there be an institutionally recognized right to die for terminally ill patients? This chapter presents reasons for doubt. When a dying patient is given the right to terminate his life, he becomes responsible for exercising or failing to exercise that option. In some circumstances, this can harm the dying patient. The chapter concludes that while there may be cases where physicians are morally justified in giving their patients the option to die, the case for an institutionally protected right to die has not yet been made.

Chapter Four

Over the past twenty-five years, palliative care medicine has offered valuable comfort to dying patients. The success of palliative care medicine, however, should be celebrated with a measure of caution. This chapter argues that the success of palliative care medicine has contributed to the emergence of a set of attitudes among end-of-life practitioners that is termed "palliative care triumphalism." Left unexamined, these attitudes have the potential to become yet another way for clinicians to avoid dealing with the reality and imminence of their patients' death.

Chapter Five

Patients who die in the clinic frequently suffer from varying forms of mental illness. Focusing on depression and schizophrenia in particular, this chapter discusses how these illnesses can impair the cognitive abilities necessary for autonomous agency. The presence of these impairments greatly complicates the clinical task of providing dying patients with appropriate medical care while respecting their right to refuse treatment. The chapter notes that judgments of decision-making capacity are often informed by ethical as well as clinical considerations.

Chapter Six

Old age and terminal illness bring special and challenges—such as the loss of independence, the progressive loss of mental and physical functioning, and the loss of a secure sense of self. This chapter introduces the idea of "comprehensive assessment" for treating the elderly and the dying. Comprehensive assessment is based on the idea that without a full understanding of the patient, one that includes cultural and social needs as well as medical facts, it is not possible to develop an optimal plan of care for the patient.

Chapter Seven

The therapeutic imperative is often misapplied at the end of life. The provision of adequate treatment is wrongly understood to require maximizing the life expectancy of dying patients. This chapter identifies several reasons for this development. After critically discussing these reasons, the chapter argues for the need to develop a consensus on the value of mortal life to justify limiting interventions in the face of approaching death.

Chapter Eight

Newly deceased patients are often used for purposes of medical training. This chapter argues that while this practice is not *per se* unethical, it can become unethical if it uses the deceased person in a way that he or she would have considered disrespectful. The chapter notes that respectful treatment of corpses varies considerably between cultures.

Index

About the Contributors

David Barnard, Ph.D., is the director of palliative care education and professor of medicine at the University of Pittsburgh. He has published and lectured extensively on ethical issues at the end of life; suffering, meaning, and hope; hospice and palliative care; and medical education.

Celia Berdes, Ph.D., is an assistant professor of medicine at Northwestern University's Buehler Center on Aging, part of the Feinberg School of Medicine.

James L. Bernat, M.D., is a professor of medicine (neurology), associate chief in the neurology section, and the director of the Program in Clinical Ethics at Dartmouth College School of Medicine. Dr. Bernat has published extensively on the ethical issues at the end of life. He received his M.D. from Cornell University.

Linda Emanuel, M.D., Ph.D., is the Buehler Professor of Medicine and director of the Buehler Center on Aging at the Feinberg School of Medicine and the health section director of the Ford Motor Company Center on Global Citizenship at the Kellogg School of Management at Northwestern University. She is the founder and principal of the national Education for Physicians in End-of-Life Care (EPEC).

Robert Fogerty is a former student of Dr. John Paris and is presently a first-year medical student at Northwestern Medical School.

Linda Ganzini, M.D., is the director of the Palliative Care Fellowship at the Portland VA Medical Center and professor of psychiatry in the Oregon Health & Science University School of Medicine.

Elizabeth R. Goy, Ph.D., is assistant professor in the Department of Psychiatry at Oregon Health & Science University and in the Mental Health Division of the Portland VA Medical Center.

Lynn A. Jansen, Ph.D., is assistant research professor of medicine at New York Medical College and assistant director of the Bioethics Institute at New York Medical College. She is also a senior medical ethicist at St. Vincent's Hospital Manhattan.

David J. Mayo, Ph.D., is a professor in the Department of Philosophy at the University of Minnesota, Duluth, and a faculty associate at the university's Center for Bioethics. He has served on the boards of directors of the American Association of Suicidology, the Midwest Chapter of the Hemlock Society, and the Death with Dignity National Center.

John J. Paris, S.J., is the Walsh Professor of Bioethics in the Department of Theology at Boston College. He has served as a consultant to the President's Commission for the Study of Ethics in Medicine, the United States Senate Committee on Aging, and the Congressional Office of Technology Assessment.

Michael D. Schreiber, M.D., is a professor of pediatrics at the University of Chicago and the associate fellowship director in the Department of Neonatology at the University of Chicago Hospital.

J. David Velleman, Ph.D., is a professor of philosophy at the University of Michigan, Ann Arbor. His research interests include ethics and moral psychology.

Mark R. Wicclair, Ph.D., is a professor of philosophy and an adjunct professor of community medicine at West Virginia University, where he has won five awards for outstanding research, teaching, and public service.